SEVEN PROVEN PRINCIPLES FOR A HAPPY MARRIAGE.

BY

DIANE T. WEE

ABOUT THE AUTHOR

Diane T. Wee is a well-known relationship specialist, author, and speaker with more than 20 years of experience assisting couples in cultivating meaningful and long-lasting marriages. Diane has dedicated her career to understanding the complexities of human connection and intimate relationship dynamics, drawing on considerable research and real-world experience.

Diane has a master's degree in marriage and family therapy and is a certified relationship coach. Through her workshops and seminars, she has led numerous couples through the obstacles of marriage, giving them with practical skills and insights to better their relationships. Her sympathetic approach promotes open communication, mutual respect, and emotional closeness, allowing couples to manage the difficulties of their relationships with confidence and compassion.

In addition to her work with couples, Diane is a popular speaker at conferences and gatherings, where she shares her knowledge of relationship development and conflict resolution. Her enthusiasm for promoting healthy relationships permeates her writing, which mixes research-backed ideas with relatable experiences and concrete advice.

Diane's earlier works have received recognition for their practical insights and entertaining approach, establishing her as a reliable voice in the field of relationship advice. Diane's latest book, *7 Proven concepts for Happy Marriages,* distills her extensive experience into seven important concepts that enable couples to form and maintain joyful, long-lasting relationships.

When Diane is not writing or working with couples, she enjoys spending time with her family, traveling, and learning about new cultures. She believes that love is a journey that takes devotion and effort, and she is dedicated to guiding couples on that journey with optimism and excitement.

COPYRIGHT

except in the case of brief quotations embodied in critical reviews and certain other noncommercial uses permitted by copyright law. For permission requests, write to the publisher at the address below.

Published by [Diane T. Wee].

This is a work of nonfiction. While best efforts have been made to ensure accuracy, the author assumes no responsibility for errors or omissions.

Table Of Contents

INTRODUCTION

The Foundation of a Happy Marriage.

Marriage, at its core, is the ultimate partnership, a pledge to walk through life together, no matter what comes your way. However, unlike in fairy tales, when "happily ever after" appears to happen effortlessly, real-life marriages are a complex mix of emotions, obstacles, and delights. They need considerably more than love to thrive. They need thought, effort, and, most importantly, a thorough grasp of what makes a marriage succeed.

Many people approach marriage with optimism, enthusiasm, and real feelings for their partner. However, as time passes, the realities of daily life become apparent, and couples frequently struggle to preserve the closeness and harmony they previously enjoyed. What begins with passion and the thrill of companionship can, if not fostered, be worn down by misunderstandings, stress, or just the passage of time. However, a happy and lasting marriage is not a myth. It is erected, piece by piece, on solid foundations.

So, what constitutes the cornerstone of a happy marriage? It goes well beyond common interests, complementary personalities, or even the depth of romantic love. It is a set of guiding principles and practices that, when followed, enable couples to deepen their bond, effectively settle disagreements, and maintain joy through life's ups and downs.

A happy marriage needs a commitment to progress, both individually and jointly. This does not imply that the journey will always be smooth or that all conflict can be avoided. Every couple experiences conflicts, frustrations, and disappointment. The crucial distinction in a happy marriage is how these obstacles are addressed. It's about realizing that marriage is a dynamic, ever-changing relationship that strengthens with conscious work and the correct tools.

Why this book?

This book does not offer fast fixes or superficial solutions. It's about tried-and-true concepts based on decades of research, real-world observations, and the experiences of many couples. These ideas are not magical, but when followed consistently, they have the potential to transform any marriage.

Why emphasis on principles? Because, while each partnership is unique, the basic requirements of a relationship are universal. We all require affection, trust, respect, and emotional support. These are the foundations of a happy marriage, and the seven concepts described in this book are intended to cultivate these important parts of your partnership.

These principles are more than just ideas; they are actionable activities you and your partner can take to create or rebuild a solid, long-lasting bond. You will learn how to communicate more effectively, how to lean toward each other during stressful times instead of pushing apart, and how to resolve problems in ways that build rather than hurt your relationship.

The Reality of Marriage

Before delving into these ideas, it's critical to realize one basic fact: no marriage is flawless. Every relationship, regardless of how in love they are, will experience difficulties. There will be moments of conflict, doubt, and times when the daily grind appears to eclipse the joy of the relationship. This is normal. The goal is not to establish a conflict-free marriage, but rather to construct one that is resilient to adversity through patience, understanding, and mutual respect.

In a happy marriage, couples learn to view dispute as an opportunity for progress rather than failure. They don't avoid difficult conversations or pretend everything is always perfect. Instead, they approach challenging situations with empathy and a desire to better understand one another. This is when emotional intelligence and availability come into play. Both are essential components of a great marriage, and will be discussed throughout this book.

Another key feature of marriage is the ability to retain affection and admiration for one another throughout time. It's easy to develop feelings for your partner in the early stages of a relationship because they're new and exciting, and you see them through an idealistic lens. However, as time passes, life comes stress, responsibilities, and obstacles that might overshadow that first admiration. Happy couples actively endeavor to maintain and strengthen their love for one another, frequently expressing gratitude, appreciation, and affection.

Developing Emotional and Practical Strength
As you work through the seven concepts in this book, you will see a harmony between the emotional and practical elements of marriage. Both are crucial. On the emotional side, you will find values that emphasize trust, empathy, and understanding. These are the essential components of a happy marriage: partners who feel sincerely heard, respected, and appreciated.

On the practical side, you'll learn ideas to help you navigate common marriage issues including dispute resolution, decision-making, and managing opposing viewpoints. Learning how to deal with everyday situations constructively is critical for long-term peace and harmony.

Furthermore, a strong marriage is one in which both parties believe they are part of something greater than themselves. This is referred to as shared meaning—the sense that you are all striving toward the same aims, values, and dreams. Whether it's raising a kid, establishing a career, or simply creating a loving and respectful household, shared meaning is what gives marriage its deeper purpose.

Why Do These Principles Matter?
The seven principles discussed in this book are more than just theoretical ideas. They are based on decades of research by relationship experts, including prominent psychologists and marriage therapists. These ideas have repeatedly demonstrated to be effective across a diverse spectrum of spouses, backgrounds, and circumstances.

By adhering to these concepts, you will learn to:
- Increase emotional intimacy: Strengthen your bond and deepen your understanding of one another.
- Manage conflict effectively by approaching conflicts in a way that leads to resolution rather than animosity.
- Maintain respect and appreciation. Even when things are bad, keep the love and admiration alive.

- Create a shared meaning. Establish a sense of purpose and direction in your relationship.

Whether you're newlyweds or have been married for decades, these principles provide a framework for developing and maintaining a successful, happy marriage.

Your journey begins here.

Marriage is a lifelong adventure that, like any other, involves planning, dedication, and a willingness to learn along the way. As you embark on this journey with your partner, remember that the basis of a happy marriage is not something you construct once and then forget about. It is a structure that must be maintained, strengthened, and sometimes completely rebuilt.

In the following pages, you'll learn about each of the seven principles in depth, as well as practical guidance and real-life examples of how they've helped couples like you. Take your time, consider how these concepts apply to your own marriage, and be open to the process of change. With time, work, and the correct tools, you can create the marriage of your dreams—one full of love, respect, joy, and resilience.

Let us begin this trip together.

Understanding the Value of Strong Relationships

Strong relationships are the foundation of a satisfying and meaningful life. Our interactions, whether with a partner, family members, friends, or colleagues, influence who we are, how we perceive the world, and the level of satisfaction we reach. Relationships, at their core, provide us with connection, support, and a sense of belonging, all of which we naturally seek. But what defines a strong relationship, and why are they so valuable?

Emotional and Psychological Benefits
Humans are sociable beings by nature. We are born reliant on others for survival, development, and progress. Relationships provide us with emotional security—a place where we can express ourselves, be vulnerable, and get support when faced with life's obstacles. This emotional safety is critical for our general well-being.

Research regularly shows that those who maintain solid, supportive relationships are happier and healthier. These partnerships provide a shield against stress, anxiety, and despair. When we feel connected to others, our bodies create oxytocin, also known as the "love hormone." This hormone relieves tension and fosters feelings of peace and trust. In other words, meaningful connections have a significant physiologic impact on our mental health, lowering levels of the stress hormone cortisol.

Loneliness and poor connections, on the other hand, can cause mental anguish, contributing to a variety of health problems such as melancholy, anxiety, and even physical disorders like high blood pressure or weakened immune systems. The emotional toll of dysfunctional or failed relationships can be heavy, making it difficult to achieve happiness and fulfillment in life.

Building Trust and Emotional Security

Trust is fundamental to healthy partnerships. Trust is the basis upon which emotional stability rests. Without trust, it is difficult to feel safe or connected to others. This holds true in all types of relationships, but it is especially important in intimate connections. Trust enables us to be open and honest without fear of being judged or damaged. It provides us the confidence to express our most intimate ideas and feelings, knowing that we are respected and understood.

Emotional security comes from knowing that no matter what, the other person will support you. This form of support promotes resilience. When we face obstacles, whether personal or external, having someone to lean on helps us get through them more easily. In the inevitable storms of life, a healthy relationship serves as a haven, a secure harbor.

The Role of Communication

Communication is frequently regarded as the key to any successful relationship—and with good reason. How we communicate has a direct impact on the strength of our relationships. Open, honest, and respectful communication promotes understanding and connection, but bad communication can result in misunderstandings, resentment, and even confrontation.

Strong relationships are distinguished by active listening, in which one person not only hears but also sincerely attempts to grasp the perspective of the other. It's important to participate in the conversation rather than simply waiting your turn to speak. In good relationships, partners and friends do not avoid uncomfortable conversations. They approach them with care and patience, recognizing that confronting challenges directly on is critical to growth and comprehension.

In contrast, when communication fails, relationships suffer. Misunderstandings cause anger, and unresolved confrontations can linger, resulting in emotional distance. Even the strongest ties can be weakened over time. That is why learning to communicate effectively, especially during disagreements, is a critical ability for developing and sustaining healthy relationships.

Mutual respect and shared values.
Strong partnerships are founded on mutual respect. Respect entails valuing the other person's thoughts, feelings, and limits. It entails viewing them as an equal partner in the relationship, with needs and desires as essential as your own. In good relationships, respect is demonstrated via acts of compassion, consideration, and recognition of each other's worth.

Shared values are one of the defining characteristics of strong relationships. While people's hobbies and personality traits vary, having shared basic principles fosters a sense of unity and direction. These values may include common family ideas, ethics, life goals, or dispute resolution strategies. When partners or friends share similar ground in these areas, they are more likely to handle obstacles as a group rather than as individuals pulling in opposite directions.

However, strong partnerships may not require total harmony in all areas. In reality, differences can strengthen a relationship if handled with respect and inquiry. What matters most is that both sides are committed to understanding and valuing each other's points of view, even if they do not always agree.

Strong Relationships and Conflict Resolution.
No partnership is without disputes. Even in the most loving, healthy relationships, disagreement is unavoidable. What distinguishes strong relationships is how problems are resolved. Conflict does not indicate a breakdown in relationships characterized by trust, communication, and respect; rather, it represents an opportunity for progress.

In a solid relationship, both sides embrace dispute as a means of settlement rather than competition. Instead than attempting to "win" a dispute, the goal is to reach a solution that benefits both parties, or at the very least, to gain a better understanding of each other's needs. This does not imply avoiding conflict, but rather approaching it with patience and empathy.

Healthy conflict resolution entails active listening, emotional validation, and collaborative problem-solving. It's about striking a balance between being honest about one's sentiments and keeping open to the other person's point of view. When couples or friends approach dispute with mutual respect and a desire to develop their relationship, they are more likely to emerge feeling closer and more understood.

The Role of Vulnerability

Vulnerability is another important aspect of healthy partnerships. It may seem contradictory, but being vulnerable—allowing someone to see you fully, flaws and all—strengthens relationships. Indeed, vulnerability promotes closeness since it means letting go of pretense and trusting the other person with your true self.

In close relationships, vulnerability enables people to connect on a deeper level. It fosters emotional connection that surface-level encounters cannot provide. Being vulnerable, whether by discussing anxieties, acknowledging mistakes, or expressing emotion, is a brave gesture that demonstrates trust and emotional openness. When both people in a relationship are willing to be vulnerable, true intimacy can grow.

The Ripple Effect of Strong Relationships

The importance of solid relationships goes beyond the persons involved. When we have healthy, supportive relationships, it has an impact on every element of our life. People in strong relationships are more confident, resilient, and fulfilled. These characteristics permeate various aspects of life, such as employment and social interactions, as well as physical health and mental wellbeing.

Strong relationships determine how we interact with our surroundings. People who feel safe and respected in their relationships are more likely to be sympathetic, empathetic, and willing to make new connections. They're also better prepared to deal with stress and negotiate life's problems since they know they have a solid support system.

The Power of Connection

Strong relationships have immeasurable value. They are critical for our emotional well-being, psychological health, and overall happiness. A strong relationship is a source of joy, comfort, and resilience—it allows us to be ourselves while knowing we are respected and supported.

Building and maintaining solid connections takes time and intention, but the benefits are tremendous. By cultivating our relationships through trust, communication, respect, and vulnerability, we not only improve our personal well-being but also lay the groundwork for a better, more meaningful existence. Strong relationships allow us to be our best selves while also providing the love and support we need to handle life's difficulties.

Overview of the Seven Principles.

Marriage is frequently viewed as a union founded on love, but as time passes, it becomes evident that maintaining a happy and fulfilling marriage takes more than simply devotion. It takes understanding, patience, and dedication to certain guiding principles that serve as the foundation of a successful partnership. These seven principles are more than just intellectual ideals; they are practical, tried-and-true techniques for creating a long-lasting marriage that can withstand life's inevitable ups and downs.

These concepts are the outcome of decades of research into how relationships work. They provide couples with a clear road map for not just avoiding frequent errors that lead to conflict and distance, but also actively strengthening their relationship on a daily basis. Whether you're newlyweds or have been married for decades, the concepts below provide a solid foundation for building and maintaining a good marriage.

1. Enhance Your Love Maps

The first concept is to establish a strong emotional connection through profound knowledge. A "love map" is essentially a mental image of your partner's inner world, including their thoughts, emotions, hopes, dreams, and even fears. Couples with extensive love maps know each other well. They can remember their partner's preferences, dislikes, stresses, joys, and desires.

Enhancing your love maps establishes a foundation of emotional closeness. Knowing your partner on this level enables you to provide assistance during difficult times while also celebrating life's joys together. This notion encourages couples to remain curious about each other and learn new things about their partner, even after many years of marriage.

2. Develop fondness and admiration.

The second guideline emphasizes the necessity of having a good attitude toward your companion. Fondness and appreciation serve as a barrier against negativity, making it easier to deal with the unavoidable disagreements that arise in every marriage. Couples who cultivate admiration actively focus on each other's excellent qualities rather than dwelling on imperfections.

Admiration does not happen by chance. Creating a culture of respect and gratitude demands conscious effort. This idea encourages couples to express gratitude on a regular basis, to remind each other of the traits that drew them together in the first place, and to speak positively even during times of conflict. When appreciation is great, it is far more difficult for resentment to take hold.

3. Turn toward each other rather than away.
One of the most important aspects of a successful marriage is how partners respond to each other's requests for connection. These bids could be as easy as inquiring how your partner's day went, or as serious as seeking emotional assistance during a crisis. When partners continually turn toward each other and respond with interest and involvement, they develop trust and closeness.

This idea encourages couples to be emotionally available to one another and to realize the value of little, daily contacts. Turning toward your partner in these situations, rather than aside or ignoring them, strengthens your bond and maintains the partnership emotionally healthy.

4. Allow Your Partner to Influence You.
Mutual respect and an openness to influence are essential components of a happy marriage. This idea entails being willing to consider your partner's viewpoints, desires, and needs. In a healthy marriage, choices are made together, and both partners believe that their perspectives are important. It is not about power or control, but about equilibrium, cooperation, and compromise.

This principle encourages partners to be humble, open-minded, and to recognize that their partner's input is equally significant as their own. When partners allow each other to influence them, they develop a sense of equality and partnership, which enriches the whole connection.

5. Solve Your Solvable Problems.
Every couple has problems, but not all problems are the same. Some problems are manageable, while others are permanent, due to underlying personality differences. The fifth principle focuses on addressing issues that can be solved via conversation and compromise.

Solvable difficulties frequently concentrate around everyday issues such as chores, income, or parenting. Couples that handle these challenges constructively employ effective communication strategies, avoid blaming or stonewalling, and approach the matter with the objective of finding a solution that benefits both sides. Couples can lessen stress and avoid resentment by learning how to approach these issues respectfully and productively.

6. Overcome Gridlock in Ongoing Conflicts

Not all marital conflicts have simple solutions. Some arguments arise from firmly held ideals, personality traits, or unfulfilled ambitions that are difficult to reconcile. These are what relationship specialists refer to as "perpetual conflicts." While these issues may never be completely resolved, the idea is to discover strategies to manage them without jeopardizing the partnership.

This approach teaches couples how to traverse stuck issues by first comprehending the underlying meaning of the disagreement. It promotes empathy and acceptance, assisting couples in transitioning from a state of dissatisfaction to mutual respect and understanding. Recognizing that some problems will endure allows couples to learn to live with these differences in a way that does not jeopardize their relationship.

7. Create shared meaning.

A marriage is about more than just two people coexisting; it is about building a life together that has significance. This third concept emphasizes the necessity of creating a shared vision, rituals, objectives, and values to give your partnership a feeling of purpose and direction.

Couples who generate shared meaning establish traditions, long-term goals, and a feeling of purpose that transcends the mundane. Whether it's raising a family, supporting each other's aspirations, or creating a home full of love and laughter, shared purpose fosters a stronger sense of connection. It makes couples feel like they're a part of something bigger than themselves, giving their relationship a deep feeling of purpose.

The seven concepts mentioned here form a thorough foundation for creating a happy, long-lasting marriage. They are not fast fixes, but rather long-term methods requiring deliberate effort, patience, and a real desire to progress. Couples can build a healthy and durable relationship by increasing emotional connection, retaining appreciation, leaning toward each other, and handling problems with respect.

Marriage is a journey, and these ideas help to guide you along the road. Whether you're facing hardships or simply want to enhance your bond, following these principles can help you create a relationship that not only survives but flourishes, full with love, trust, and long-lasting satisfaction.

Chapter 1: Enhance Your Love Maps

Every strong marriage is built on a deep emotional connection that goes beyond everyday routines and surface-level encounters. This emotional link begins with a basic grasp of each other's inner world—what makes your spouse tick, their dreams, their fears, and even the seemingly minor elements that define who they are. This is what relationship specialists call "love maps."

A love map is a mental representation of your partner's emotional geography. It covers all you know about them—their likes and dislikes, the names of their closest friends, their key life goals, and their main concerns. Essentially, it's about getting to know your partner as deeply as possible and keeping connected as you both grow throughout time.

Why Do Love Maps Matter?
You may question why such detailed knowledge is required. Isn't love enough? The answer is "no." While love is a tremendous force, it cannot sustain a marriage indefinitely. Relationships are based on connection, which comes from understanding. When you know your spouse well, you can provide the support, love, and comfort they require—especially during difficult times.

Consider the following scenario: one spouse is anxious about work, while the other is oblivious of the severity of the situation. Without this understanding, the stressed partner may feel isolated or unsupported, resulting in emotional distance. On the other hand, knowing what's going on in your partner's life allows you to respond in ways that build your bond—whether it's delivering a soothing word, taking on extra domestic responsibilities to alleviate their stress, or simply being present to listen.

Love maps are also important during times of strife. When arguments emerge, couples with strong love maps may handle them with more empathy and compassion. They don't just dispute about the subject; they also comprehend the underlying emotions that are causing the conflict. This greater understanding can help de-escalate arguments and keep both partners feeling heard, even if they disagree.

How to Improve Your Love Maps
Creating and improving love maps is a continual process. It is not something you do once and then forget about. To keep in tune with your partner's changing wants, desires, and concerns, you must instead be curious, attentive, and make a deliberate effort.

Here are some strategies to improve your love map:

1. Ask questions—and keep asking them
Asking questions is one of the simplest and most effective ways to create a love map. Become curious about your partner's world. Inquire about their dreams, fears, and everyday experiences. Here are some examples of questions that can help you better understand:

- What are you currently passionate about or working on in your personal life or career?
- What is the source of your greatest anxiety right now?
- Are you considering pursuing any new objectives or hobbies?
- How do you feel about where our relationship is going?

- What have you always wanted to do but haven't had the opportunity?

These kinds of questions aren't only for newlyweds; they're also vital for long-term couples. People adapt, grow, and evolve, and it's critical to stay current on how your partner's ambitions and concerns alter over time.

2. Be attentive and observant.
Your partner may not always express how they feel or think. This is why it's critical to be aware of their behavior, body language, and mood. Is your partner more withdrawn than usual? Are they excited about something but haven't shared it yet? Take note of these small cues and check in with them.

Observation extends beyond recognizing when something is incorrect. It also entails paying attention to the things that make people happy or comfortable. Knowing that your partner enjoys their coffee in a particular way or that they unwind by listening to a specific podcast may appear insignificant, but these simple things are what contribute to a stronger sense of connection.

3. Make Time for Regular Check-ins.
Life becomes busy, and it's easy to go days or weeks without truly connecting with your partner on a deeper level. Here's where regular check-ins come in. Set aside time each day, even if it is only 10 or 15 minutes, to discuss topics other than logistics or daily activities. Use this opportunity to inquire

about how they are feeling, what has been on their mind, and any recent happenings in their lives that they would like to discuss.

These check-ins do not need to be official, sit-down discussions. They can happen when you're walking, eating dinner, or even winding down before bedtime. The goal is to stay in sync with each other's emotional world, which helps to prevent emotional drift over time.

4. Celebrate Your Partner's Wins—Big and Small

Part of building a strong love map is actively participating in your partner's life, which includes celebrating their accomplishments, no matter how small. Whether they've achieved a major milestone at work or successfully completed a personal goal, acknowledging these moments builds closeness.

When your partner feels seen and celebrated, it reinforces the idea that you're not just living parallel lives but truly sharing the journey together. This helps create a strong emotional bond that serves as the foundation for a healthy and happy marriage

Love Maps in Everyday Life

The concept of love maps may seem abstract at first, but it plays out in everyday life in simple yet meaningful ways. For example, if you know that your partner has a presentation coming up at work that they're nervous about, you can offer them encouragement in advance and check in afterward to see how it went. These small actions—based on your knowledge of what's important to them—strengthen your connection.

Similarly, understanding your partner's deeper emotional needs can help you offer support in more tailored ways. For example, if your partner tends to shut down when they're feeling overwhelmed, knowing this can help you approach them with patience and care, rather than frustration.

Over time, as you continually update your love map, you build a more resilient and understanding relationship. You'll be able to anticipate each other's needs, respond to stress with greater empathy, and ultimately, maintain a closer emotional connection.

The Payoff of Enhanced Love Maps
Couples with strong love maps report feeling more satisfied in their marriages and better equipped to handle life's challenges. When you truly know your partner—when you're attuned to their thoughts, feelings, and desires—it becomes easier to navigate both the joyful and difficult times in life together. You become a team that works in harmony, with a shared understanding of what makes each other tick.

In contrast, when love maps are weak, couples may feel disconnected or out of touch with each other's needs. This can lead to misunderstandings, frustration, and emotional distance. By investing the time and effort to enhance your love map, you're essentially investing in the long-term health and happiness of your marriage.

Enhancing your love maps is one of the most effective ways to build emotional intimacy and ensure that your relationship remains strong and connected. By staying curious, asking meaningful questions, and paying attention to your partner's emotional world, you create a solid foundation for your marriage to thrive.

This principle may seem simple, but its impact is profound. Couples who know each other deeply are better equipped to navigate life's challenges together, and they experience a deeper, more meaningful connection. So, whether you're just starting out in your marriage or have been together for many years, continually enhancing your love maps will help keep the love and intimacy alive.

Creating a Deep Emotional Connection

At the core of every fulfilling and lasting relationship is a deep emotional connection—a bond that goes beyond the superficial and taps into the very essence of what makes us human. This kind of connection doesn't just happen overnight; it's cultivated over time through mutual understanding, vulnerability, and genuine effort from both partners. While physical attraction and shared interests can bring two people together, it is the emotional connection that keeps them strong and resilient through life's challenges.

What Is a Deep Emotional Connection?

A deep emotional connection is the feeling that you truly understand your partner, and in turn, they understand you. It's the sense of being seen, heard, and valued for who you are, without pretense or judgment. When a couple has this type of bond, they can communicate on an intuitive level, often without words. It's that feeling of security and trust, knowing that your partner is there for you, not just physically but emotionally as well.

This connection is built on empathy, mutual respect, and a shared sense of purpose. It allows partners to be vulnerable with each other, to share their fears, insecurities, and hopes without fear of being misunderstood or rejected. And while it may sound lofty, creating and maintaining this kind of connection is both possible and necessary for a thriving relationship.

Why Is Emotional Connection So Important?
Without emotional connection, relationships can feel hollow, transactional, or even robotic. People in emotionally disconnected marriages often describe feeling lonely, even when they're physically together. They may go through the motions of daily life—sharing a home, raising children, or handling finances—but there's a lack of intimacy and closeness. Over time, this emotional distance can lead to feelings of resentment, frustration, or even hopelessness.

A deep emotional connection is what keeps love alive. It's the fuel that allows couples to weather conflicts, overcome life's obstacles, and continue growing together rather than apart. When both partners feel emotionally connected, they are more likely to feel satisfied in their relationship, more resilient in the face of challenges, and more committed to making their partnership work.

How to Build a Deep Emotional Connection

Building a deep emotional connection is an ongoing process. It's not something that happens automatically or stays intact without effort. Like tending to a garden, this connection needs nurturing, attention, and care. Here are some practical ways to strengthen and deepen the emotional bond with your partner:

1. Practice Active Listening

One of the most powerful ways to create a deep emotional connection is by truly listening to your partner. This means more than just hearing their words; it means listening with intent and empathy. Active listening involves giving your partner your full attention, without distractions like your phone or TV, and responding thoughtfully.

When your partner feels heard, they feel valued. It signals to them that their thoughts and feelings matter, which fosters trust and closeness. Active listening also means asking questions, seeking to understand their perspective, and validating their emotions, even if you don't necessarily agree with everything they say.

2. Be Vulnerable

Vulnerability is the cornerstone of emotional connection. It's about opening yourself up, even when it feels uncomfortable or risky. When you allow yourself to be vulnerable with your partner, you invite them into your inner world—your fears, insecurities, dreams, and hopes. This openness creates a space for deep emotional intimacy.

It's important to remember that vulnerability is a two-way street. Both partners need to feel safe enough to share their true selves without fear of judgment or rejection. This kind of trust takes time to build, but the more you practice being open and honest with each other, the deeper your emotional connection will grow.

3. Engage in Meaningful Conversations

While casual conversations about work or daily chores are important, they don't often lead to deep emotional bonding. To truly connect with your partner, you need to engage in meaningful conversations—discussions that touch on your deeper thoughts, feelings, and experiences.

Talk about your dreams for the future, your values, and what gives you a sense of purpose. Share your fears, the things that keep you up at night, and the moments in life that have shaped you. These types of conversations create a profound understanding of who your partner is at their core and allow you to connect on a deeper emotional level.

4. Show Empathy and Compassion

Empathy—the ability to understand and share the feelings of another—is a crucial component of emotional connection. When your partner is going through a tough time, showing empathy allows them to feel understood and supported. It's not just about offering solutions; often, it's about being present, offering a shoulder to lean on, and saying, "I'm here for you."

Compassion goes hand in hand with empathy. It's the active expression of your care and concern for your partner. This might mean doing something kind for them when they're having a hard day, or simply offering words of encouragement and love. These gestures, while seemingly small, go a long way in building and maintaining emotional intimacy.

5. Prioritize Quality Time Together
In the busyness of everyday life, it's easy for couples to drift apart emotionally. Work, kids, and other responsibilities can often take precedence, leaving little time for connection. However, spending quality time together is essential for keeping the emotional bond strong.

Quality time doesn't necessarily mean grand gestures or elaborate date nights. It's about being fully present with each other, whether that's during a quiet dinner at home, a walk in the park, or even just sitting together and talking. The key is to carve out time where you can focus on each other without distractions, allowing space for conversation, affection, and reconnection.

6. Express Love and Appreciation Regularly
Sometimes, we assume our partner knows how much we love and appreciate them, but saying it out loud is incredibly important. Regularly expressing love and appreciation

strengthens the emotional connection by reinforcing positive feelings in the relationship.

Tell your partner what you admire about them. Acknowledge the things they do that make you feel loved. Small, consistent expressions of gratitude and affection—whether through words, actions, or gestures—help to keep the emotional bond alive and thriving.

7. Work Through Conflict with Respect

Every couple experiences conflict, but how you handle those conflicts can either deepen or damage your emotional connection. Instead of viewing disagreements as a battle to be won, approach them with respect and a desire to understand each other's perspective.

During arguments, try to stay calm and avoid saying hurtful things in the heat of the moment. Listen to your partner's concerns and express your own feelings without placing blame. Couples who resolve conflicts with empathy and respect are able to maintain and even strengthen their emotional connection over time.

The Benefits of a Deep Emotional Connection

When you and your partner have a strong emotional connection, everything else in the relationship tends to fall into place. You're more likely to feel satisfied and fulfilled in the relationship, and you'll have an easier time navigating challenges together. Here are some key benefits of a deep emotional bond:

- **Increased Trust:** With emotional intimacy comes trust. You trust that your partner has your back, and you feel secure in knowing that you're both committed to the relationship.

- **Better Communication:** Emotional connection leads to open, honest communication. When you're emotionally close, you're more likely to share your thoughts and feelings without fear of judgment.

- **Greater Resilience:** Couples with a deep emotional connection are better equipped to handle stress and conflict. Their bond acts as a buffer against the challenges life throws their way.

- **Lasting Happiness**: Ultimately, a deep emotional connection is one of the greatest predictors of long-term relationship satisfaction. Couples who feel emotionally connected tend to be happier, more affectionate, and more committed to each other over time.

Creating and maintaining a deep emotional connection requires effort, vulnerability, and genuine care. It's about continually learning, growing, and evolving with your partner, while also providing them with a sense of security and support. The emotional bond you build together will become the foundation of your relationship, helping you navigate life's highs and lows with love and understanding. When both partners are committed to nurturing this connection, it becomes the key to a truly fulfilling and lasting partnership.

Strategies to Understand Each Other's Inner Worlds

One of the most critical aspects of a successful marriage or long-term relationship is understanding your partner on a deep, emotional level—what relationship experts often call knowing each other's "inner worlds." This goes beyond knowing their favorite color or preferred food; it's about understanding what makes your partner tick, their hopes, fears, insecurities, and dreams. This intimate knowledge strengthens the emotional bond and creates a foundation of trust, empathy, and mutual respect. The deeper you understand each other, the more resilient your relationship becomes.

Understanding your partner's inner world is not something that happens naturally; it requires intentional effort. It's an ongoing process that evolves as each person grows and changes over time. Below are several strategies you can use to deepen your knowledge of your partner's inner world and, in turn, create a stronger, more connected relationship.

1. Ask Open-Ended Questions

The first step to understanding your partner's inner world is to ask meaningful questions—questions that go beyond the surface and invite deeper conversations. Open-ended questions encourage your partner to reflect on their thoughts, feelings, and experiences, giving you a window into their inner life. These types of questions can't be answered with a simple "yes" or "no"; they require thought and often lead to revealing insights.

Here are some examples of open-ended questions:

- "What's something that has been on your mind lately?"
- "What are your biggest dreams for the future?"
- "What is something that makes you feel truly happy?"
- "What are some things that stress you out, and how can I help ease that stress?"
- "Is there anything you've been wanting to talk about but haven't had the chance to?"

These questions create opportunities for deeper connection, allowing you to learn more about your partner's emotional landscape, current worries, and desires.

2. Be Curious, Not Judgmental

Asking questions is just the beginning. When your partner opens up, it's crucial that you approach their answers with curiosity and empathy, not judgment. People often hesitate to share their true thoughts and feelings if they fear being criticized, dismissed, or misunderstood. To create a safe space for your partner to be vulnerable, listen without jumping to conclusions or offering solutions right away.

For example, if your partner shares a fear or insecurity, avoid responding with, "That's silly, you shouldn't feel that way." Instead, try something like, "I can understand why you'd feel that way. Can you tell me more about what's been going on?"

This approach shows that you respect their feelings and are genuinely interested in understanding their perspective.

3. Practice Active Listening

Active listening is an essential skill for truly understanding your partner's inner world. It involves giving your full attention to what your partner is saying—without distractions or interruptions—and responding in a way that shows you're engaged and empathetic.

To practice active listening:

Make eye contact and put away distractions like your phone or the TV.

Nod or offer verbal affirmations like "I see" or "That makes sense" to show you're following along.

Repeat or paraphrase what your partner has said to ensure you understand correctly. For example, "It sounds like you're feeling overwhelmed by work lately."

Ask follow-up questions to dive deeper into their thoughts and feelings, such as, "How long have you been feeling this way?" or "What can I do to support you through this?"

By actively listening, you show your partner that their inner world matters to you and that you value their thoughts and feelings.

4. Create a Judgment-Free Space for Sharing

Emotional vulnerability thrives in an environment of safety and trust. If you want your partner to feel comfortable sharing their deepest thoughts and emotions, it's essential to create a judgment-free space where they know they can be honest without fear of criticism or rejection.

Here are a few ways to foster this kind of environment:
- Stay calm during difficult conversations. If your partner shares something that surprises or upsets you, try to stay composed and avoid reacting impulsively.
- Encourage openness. Let your partner know that you're always available to listen and that there's no topic too small or too uncomfortable to discuss.
- Validate their feelings. Even if you don't fully agree with what they're saying, it's important to acknowledge their feelings as valid. For example, "I can see why you feel hurt by that," or "It sounds like you've been carrying a lot of stress."

When your partner feels emotionally safe with you, they'll be more likely to open up about their inner world, knowing that they won't be judged for their thoughts or feelings.

5. Engage in Regular Emotional Check-Ins

Life can get busy, and it's easy to fall into the trap of talking only about surface-level topics, like work schedules or household chores. However, maintaining a strong emotional connection requires making time for deeper conversations. Regular emotional check-ins are an excellent way to stay in touch with each other's inner worlds.

Schedule regular moments—whether it's weekly or even daily—where you can sit down together and talk about how you're feeling. These check-ins don't have to be formal or lengthy; they can happen over dinner, during a walk, or before bed. The key is to make a habit of asking each other, "How are you really feeling?" or "What's been on your mind lately?"

During these check-ins, you can:
- Share your highs and lows from the week.
- Discuss any worries or stressors.
- Talk about personal goals and how you're feeling about them.
- Express gratitude for each other or acknowledge ways you've felt supported recently.

These regular moments of connection help keep both partners on the same emotional page and prevent feelings of disconnection from building up over time.

6. Respect and Support Each Other's Individuality

Understanding your partner's inner world also means recognizing that they are a unique individual with their own needs, desires, and goals. While you share many aspects of your lives, it's important to support each other's personal growth and individuality. Encourage your partner to pursue their passions, hobbies, or career aspirations, even if they don't directly involve you.

Supporting each other's independence shows respect for the other person's individuality and demonstrates that you are invested in their happiness and well-being. This mutual respect strengthens the bond between you and deepens your understanding of each other's inner worlds.

7. Be Patient and Persistent

Understanding your partner's inner world is not a one-time event; it's an ongoing process that evolves over time. People change, and their inner worlds shift as they grow and encounter new experiences. Be patient with this process and persistent in your efforts to understand your partner. Don't get discouraged if they're not immediately forthcoming or if it takes time to uncover deeper layers of their emotional life.

Sometimes, life's challenges—stress, fatigue, or external pressures—can make it harder for your partner to open up. Be patient and continue showing up for them with empathy and curiosity. Over time, they'll feel more comfortable sharing their inner world with you.

8. Celebrate Their Wins and Support Their Struggles

Another important aspect of understanding your partner's inner world is being present for both the good and the bad. Celebrate their accomplishments and milestones, no matter how big or small. Acknowledge their hard work and cheer them on in their successes.

Equally, be there for them during times of struggle or hardship. Offer a listening ear, a shoulder to cry on, or just quiet support when they need it most. Being emotionally present during both the highs and lows of life strengthens your bond and shows that you're invested in their well-being.

Understanding each other's inner worlds is one of the most powerful ways to create a strong, emotionally fulfilling relationship. It requires consistent effort, open communication, and a willingness to be vulnerable. By practicing empathy, asking meaningful questions, and creating a safe space for sharing, you and your partner can build a deep emotional connection that will not only sustain your relationship but also help it thrive over time.

Chapter 2: Develop Fondness and Admiration

At the heart of every strong and happy relationship lies a foundation of mutual fondness and admiration. These feelings are what keep couples bonded over time, allowing them to appreciate each other's positive qualities even in the face of inevitable challenges. Fondness and admiration are not just about liking or being attracted to your partner; they are deeper emotions rooted in respect, appreciation, and a genuine affection for who the other person is. Developing and maintaining these feelings is essential for creating a lasting and fulfilling partnership.

When fondness and admiration are strong, they act as a buffer against conflict and negativity. In contrast, when these emotions are neglected or begin to fade, the relationship can become vulnerable to resentment, frustration, and emotional distance. Fortunately, there are intentional strategies couples can use to cultivate and nurture these positive emotions, ensuring they remain a constant in the relationship.

The Importance of Fondness and Admiration
Fondness and admiration are often described as the "antidote" to contempt and negativity. In many struggling relationships, partners begin to lose sight of each other's positive qualities, focusing instead on flaws, annoyances, or mistakes. When this happens, it becomes easier to harbor feelings of resentment or contempt, which can slowly erode the relationship's foundation.

However, when partners consciously cultivate fondness and admiration, they create an emotional safety net that helps them weather difficult times. These feelings remind both partners of why they fell in love in the first place and help them focus on the positive aspects of their relationship, even when things aren't going perfectly.

Fondness and admiration help partners maintain a sense of emotional closeness and connection. They encourage each person to look for the good in their partner, reinforcing positive behavior and strengthening the bond between them. Couples who actively nurture these feelings are more likely to feel satisfied in their relationship and are better equipped to handle conflicts constructively.

Strategies for Developing Fondness and Admiration
Maintaining fondness and admiration requires effort and intention, but the good news is that these feelings can be cultivated, even in relationships that have become strained or distant. Here are several strategies to help you and your partner develop and strengthen these essential emotions.

1. Reflect on Positive Memories
One of the simplest and most effective ways to reignite feelings of fondness and admiration is to reflect on positive memories from your relationship. Take time to reminisce about the moments that made you fall in love—whether it's your first date, an unforgettable trip, or a time when your partner showed kindness or support during a challenging situation.

By focusing on these positive experiences, you can reconnect with the feelings of warmth and affection that initially drew you to your partner. Try asking each other questions like:

- "What is one of your favorite memories from when we first started dating?"
- "What was a moment when you felt especially proud of us as a couple?"
- "Can you think of a time when I did something that made you feel really loved or appreciated?"

These conversations help bring those positive memories to the forefront, reminding both partners of the strengths in their relationship.

2. Express Appreciation Regularly

Showing appreciation is one of the most powerful ways to keep fondness and admiration alive. It's easy to take your partner for granted over time, especially when life gets busy with work, children, or other responsibilities. However, taking the time to express gratitude for the small things your partner does—whether it's making dinner, offering emotional support, or simply being a good listener—can have a profound impact on your relationship.

Here are a few simple ways to express appreciation:

- Say thank you for the little things, like making the bed, picking up groceries, or being there when you needed to vent after a tough day.
- Acknowledge effort. Even if your partner didn't get something exactly right, recognizing their effort shows that you appreciate their intentions.

- Compliment your partner often. Let them know what you admire about them, whether it's their sense of humor, their work ethic, or their kindness.

Expressing appreciation regularly not only reinforces your partner's positive behavior but also helps you focus on their good qualities, fostering deeper feelings of admiration.

3. Celebrate Each Other's Successes

One of the hallmarks of a healthy relationship is the ability to genuinely celebrate each other's successes. Whether it's a big promotion at work, achieving a personal goal, or even mastering a new hobby, taking the time to acknowledge and celebrate these accomplishments fosters a sense of mutual admiration and support.

When your partner achieves something, make an effort to show how proud you are. Celebrate their success with words of encouragement, a special dinner, or a simple gesture that shows you're rooting for them. Celebrating each other's achievements, no matter how big or small, reinforces the idea that you're in each other's corner and that you admire and respect what your partner brings to the relationship.

4. Focus on Your Partner's Positive Qualities

In long-term relationships, it's easy to become hyper-aware of your partner's flaws or quirks that may annoy you over time. However, choosing to focus on your partner's positive qualities can help keep feelings of fondness and admiration alive. When you notice something you love or admire about your partner, make a mental note of it or, better yet, share it with them.

For example, if you admire your partner's patience, generosity, or sense of humor, make an effort to acknowledge those traits regularly. By focusing on what you appreciate about your partner, you reinforce positive feelings and build a more resilient emotional connection.

5. Build a Culture of Respect

Respect is the cornerstone of admiration. Without mutual respect, it's difficult to maintain feelings of fondness, especially during times of conflict. Building a culture of respect within your relationship means treating each other with kindness, even when you disagree or are upset.

Here are a few ways to foster respect in your relationship:
- Listen without interrupting when your partner is speaking, and show that you value their thoughts and feelings, even if you don't always agree.
- Avoid sarcasm, criticism, or contempt during arguments. Instead, try to approach disagreements with empathy and a desire to understand each other's perspectives.
- Honor your partner's boundaries and needs, showing that you respect their individuality and personal space.

When respect is at the core of your relationship, admiration naturally follows. Both partners feel valued, heard, and supported, which strengthens the emotional bond.

6. Revisit Your Love Story

Every couple has a unique love story, and revisiting it can help rekindle feelings of admiration and fondness. Take some time to reflect on how your relationship began—what drew you to each other, the challenges you overcame, and the milestones you've achieved together. These memories serve as a reminder of the love, admiration, and respect that has been present from the start.

Consider activities like:
- Looking through old photos or letters from when you first started dating.
- Talking about your first impressions of each other and what qualities you found most attractive.
- Reflecting on how your relationship has grown and how you've both evolved as individuals and as a couple.

Revisiting your love story helps bring back those early feelings of excitement, admiration, and affection, reinforcing the positive emotions that keep your relationship strong.

7. Be Kind and Affectionate Daily

Acts of kindness and affection are small but powerful ways to express fondness and admiration in your everyday interactions. Simple gestures like holding hands, giving a hug, or offering a kind word can strengthen your emotional bond and keep feelings of closeness alive.

Make an effort to show affection and kindness regularly, even when life is hectic or stressful. These small moments of connection remind your partner that they are loved and appreciated, reinforcing the positive emotions that sustain a happy relationship.

Developing and maintaining fondness and admiration is one of the most important investments you can make in your relationship. These emotions create a strong foundation of mutual respect, appreciation, and affection, helping couples navigate challenges with greater resilience and positivity. By focusing on your partner's positive qualities, expressing appreciation regularly, and creating a culture of kindness and respect, you can cultivate a lasting sense of fondness and admiration that will keep your relationship thriving for years to come.

Cultivating Positive Feelings Through the Power of Respect and Appreciation

At the core of every thriving relationship are two essential qualities: respect and appreciation. These qualities not only foster positive emotions but also act as the glue that holds couples together through life's inevitable ups and downs. Without them, relationships can easily deteriorate into a cycle of misunderstandings, resentment, and emotional disconnection. However, when respect and appreciation are consciously cultivated, they have the power to transform even the most challenging relationships into harmonious and fulfilling partnerships.

Learning to cultivate positive feelings via respect and appreciation is a skill that can be developed and strengthened over time. It requires conscious effort, but the rewards—stronger emotional bonds, a deeper sense of connection, and increased relationship satisfaction—are well worth it.

The Role of Respect in Cultivating Positive Feelings

Respect is the foundation upon which all healthy relationships are built. It's more than just politeness or good manners; respect is about truly valuing your partner as an individual, honoring their thoughts, feelings, and needs, and treating them with kindness and consideration, even when you disagree or are in conflict. Respect allows both partners to feel safe, heard, and validated, creating an environment where positive feelings can flourish.

Here are a few ways respect plays a key role in cultivating positive feelings:

1. Fostering Emotional Safety

When respect is at the forefront of a relationship, it creates an environment of emotional safety. Partners know that, even during disagreements or tough times, they will be treated with care and dignity. This sense of safety allows both people to express themselves openly, without fear of judgment or rejection. Emotional safety is crucial for building trust and deepening intimacy, and it is through this trust that positive emotions like love, affection, and admiration can grow.

2. Encouraging Open Communication

Respectful communication is the backbone of any strong relationship. When partners communicate with respect, they listen to each other attentively, without interrupting or dismissing the other person's feelings. This kind of communication leads to better understanding and fewer misunderstandings, fostering a sense of connection and mutual support. When each partner feels heard and respected, positive feelings naturally follow.

3. Nurturing Individuality

Respect also means honoring each other's individuality. In a healthy relationship, both partners should feel free to pursue their own passions, interests, and goals without feeling controlled or criticized. This respect for personal space and autonomy not only strengthens the relationship but also allows both partners to grow as individuals. When partners feel supported in their personal journeys, they are more likely to feel positive and fulfilled, both within the relationship and in their own lives.

The Power of Appreciation in Strengthening Relationships
While respect lays the groundwork for emotional safety and open communication, appreciation is what keeps love and admiration alive. Expressing appreciation for your partner's actions, qualities, and contributions creates a positive feedback loop, where both people feel valued and recognized. In turn, this sense of appreciation fuels feelings of affection, gratitude, and mutual respect.

Here are some key ways appreciation can enhance positive feelings in a relationship:

1. Building Emotional Resilience

Appreciation helps build emotional resilience by shifting the focus from what's wrong to what's right. In the midst of daily stressors or relationship challenges, it's easy to dwell on your partner's flaws or the things that frustrate you. However, when you make a conscious effort to appreciate the small things your partner does—whether it's preparing your favorite meal, supporting you during a tough day, or simply being a caring presence—you begin to see them in a more positive light. This shift in perspective helps you navigate difficult times with more patience and understanding.

2. Reinforcing Positive Behavior

Appreciation is a powerful way to reinforce positive behavior in a relationship. When you express gratitude for your partner's efforts, it encourages them to continue those actions because they know they are valued. Whether it's acknowledging a kind gesture or complimenting your partner's strengths, appreciation creates a sense of positive reinforcement that strengthens the emotional bond between you.

For example, saying, "I really appreciate how you always take the time to listen to me when I've had a rough day," not only shows your partner that you value their support, but it also makes them feel good about being there for you. This mutual reinforcement of positive behaviors contributes to a more harmonious and loving relationship.

3. Creating a Culture of Gratitude

In relationships, it's easy to take each other for granted, especially when life gets busy. However, cultivating a culture of gratitude can help maintain a sense of connection and positivity, even during hectic times. By making appreciation a regular part of your relationship, you create an atmosphere where both partners feel valued and respected. Simple acts like saying "thank you" for daily tasks or expressing admiration for your partner's qualities can go a long way in fostering positive feelings and deepening your emotional connection.

Strategies to Cultivate Respect and Appreciation

Developing a habit of respect and appreciation requires mindfulness and effort, but it can be done through small, consistent actions. Here are several strategies to help you cultivate these qualities in your relationship:

1. Practice Active Listening

Active listening is a fundamental way to show respect. When your partner is speaking, give them your full attention, make eye contact, and refrain from interrupting. Ask follow-up questions to show you're engaged, and validate their feelings by acknowledging their perspective. Active listening shows your partner that you respect their thoughts and opinions, which fosters a sense of trust and emotional closeness.

2. Acknowledge Efforts, Big and Small

Take time to acknowledge the things your partner does for you and the relationship, no matter how small. Whether it's doing chores, offering emotional support, or simply being a good listener, verbalize your appreciation. This acknowledgment doesn't need to be grand or dramatic—just a simple, heartfelt "thank you" can make a significant difference in how appreciated your partner feels.

3. Focus on Strengths, Not Flaws

While it's easy to become hyper-aware of your partner's flaws, focusing on their strengths is a much more constructive approach. Make a habit of recognizing and complimenting the things your partner does well. Whether it's their kindness, patience, or sense of humor, expressing admiration for these qualities will help you maintain a positive outlook on your relationship and reinforce feelings of love and respect.

4. Create Rituals of Appreciation

Developing rituals of appreciation can help keep positive feelings alive in your relationship. These rituals could be as simple as starting or ending each day by expressing something you're grateful for about your partner. Another idea is to periodically write notes of appreciation or send a thoughtful text to remind your partner how much they mean to you. These small gestures help build a culture of gratitude and keep feelings of love and respect fresh.

5. Respect Differences

No two people are exactly alike, and differences in opinion, habits, or preferences are inevitable in any relationship. Instead of viewing these differences as a source of conflict, approach them with curiosity and respect. Understand that your partner's perspectives and experiences shape who they are, and try to appreciate their individuality. This respect for differences fosters a deeper connection and allows you to appreciate each other's unique qualities.

Respect and appreciation are the cornerstones of a healthy, happy relationship. By actively cultivating these qualities, you create an environment of emotional safety, trust, and mutual admiration. When both partners feel respected and appreciated, positive feelings like love, joy, and gratitude naturally follow. It's through these everyday acts of respect and appreciation that couples build strong, resilient relationships that can withstand life's challenges while continuing to grow in love and connection.

Chapter 3: Turn Toward Each Other

In every relationship, small moments of connection can either strengthen or weaken the bond between partners. These moments may seem insignificant on the surface, but over time, they play a critical role in determining the overall health and happiness of a relationship. Chapter 3 focuses on the importance of turning toward each other—a concept that involves responding to your partner's bids for attention, affection, or support in a positive and engaged manner.

When partners consistently turn toward each other, they create a strong emotional foundation that allows them to feel supported, understood, and loved. On the other hand, if these small opportunities for connection are repeatedly missed or ignored, the relationship can gradually drift apart, leading to feelings of loneliness and dissatisfaction.

What Does It Mean to Turn Toward Your Partner?

Turning toward your partner is all about recognizing and responding to the everyday bids for connection that occur in a relationship. A bid can be anything from a subtle gesture—like a smile or a touch—to a verbal request for attention, help, or affection. For example, when one partner says, "Look at that beautiful sunset," or asks, "Can we talk about my day?" they are making a bid for emotional connection.

How you respond to these bids can either bring you closer or create emotional distance. When you turn toward your partner, you acknowledge their bid and respond in a positive or supportive way, which strengthens the emotional bond between you. This can be as simple as showing interest, offering a kind word, or engaging in a conversation.

In contrast, when you turn away from your partner by ignoring or dismissing their bids, it creates disconnection. Over time, repeated instances of turning away can lead to frustration, resentment, and a weakened emotional bond.

The Impact of Small Moments on Relationships
In the busyness of everyday life, it's easy to overlook the importance of small moments of connection. However, these moments add up to create the overall emotional climate of a relationship. Research shows that couples who consistently turn toward each other during everyday interactions are more likely to feel satisfied and secure in their relationship. These small acts of turning toward build trust, intimacy, and a sense of partnership, all of which contribute to long-term relationship success.

Even the smallest gestures—like sharing a laugh over a joke or offering a reassuring touch—can have a profound impact. In fact, it's often these seemingly insignificant moments that determine whether a couple feels emotionally close or distant. A strong relationship is built on thousands of these micro-moments of connection.

Why Turning Toward Each Other Matters

Turning toward your partner is not just about being polite or responsive; it's about actively choosing to invest in your relationship. Here's why this concept is so important:

1. Strengthening Emotional Bonds

Every time you turn toward your partner, you reinforce the emotional bond between you. It shows that you are there for each other, not just during major life events, but in the small, everyday moments that make up the majority of life. This consistent emotional support helps both partners feel valued and understood, creating a strong foundation of trust and intimacy.

2. Building Trust and Security

When partners turn toward each other regularly, it builds a sense of trust and security in the relationship. You come to know that your partner will be there for you, whether you need emotional support, a listening ear, or just a small moment of connection. This reliability fosters a sense of safety, which is crucial for a healthy and lasting relationship.

3. Preventing Emotional Distance

Couples who fail to turn toward each other in everyday moments often experience emotional distance over time. When bids for connection go unanswered, it can create feelings of rejection or neglect. Over time, these small disconnects can accumulate, leading to frustration, resentment, and eventually a breakdown in communication and intimacy. Consistently turning toward each other helps prevent this emotional distance from developing.

4. Navigating Conflict More Effectively

Couples who regularly turn toward each other are better equipped to handle conflict when it arises. These small moments of connection build a reservoir of positive feelings and goodwill that helps couples stay emotionally connected even during disagreements. When a relationship is built on a foundation of trust and emotional closeness, it becomes easier to navigate challenges and resolve conflicts in a constructive way.

How to Turn Toward Each Other in Everyday Life

Turning toward your partner doesn't require grand gestures or major efforts. It's about being present, engaged, and responsive in the small moments that happen every day. Here are some practical strategies for turning toward your partner:

1. Be Present and Attentive

One of the simplest ways to turn toward your partner is to be fully present when they make a bid for connection. This means putting down your phone, turning away from the TV, or pausing whatever task you're working on to give them your full attention. When you show that you're genuinely interested in what your partner is saying or doing, it sends a powerful message of care and respect.

2. Respond with Empathy

When your partner makes a bid for connection, respond with empathy and understanding. Even if you can't solve their problem or meet their request right away, acknowledging their feelings and showing that you care can make a big difference. For example, if your partner expresses frustration about a stressful day at work, simply saying, "That sounds really tough. I'm here for you," can help them feel supported and understood.

3. Engage in Meaningful Conversations

Turning toward your partner isn't just about responding to bids for connection—it's also about initiating meaningful interactions. Take time each day to check in with your partner, ask how they're feeling, or share something about your own day. These conversations don't have to be deep or lengthy, but they help maintain an emotional connection.

4. Show Affection

Affectionate gestures, whether physical or verbal, are another way to turn toward your partner. A hug, a kiss, holding hands, or even a kind word can create moments of connection that strengthen your bond. Affection helps both partners feel loved and valued, reinforcing positive feelings in the relationship.

5. Celebrate Small Wins Together

Celebrate the small victories and positive moments in your partner's life. Whether it's a compliment about their work, acknowledging their efforts at home, or simply expressing gratitude for something they've done, celebrating these moments together helps foster a sense of appreciation and partnership.

6. Stay Curious About Each Other
Turning toward your partner also involves staying curious about their thoughts, feelings, and experiences. Even in long-term relationships, there is always more to learn about each other. Ask open-ended questions, share your own thoughts, and explore new topics of conversation. This curiosity keeps the relationship dynamic and helps deepen your emotional connection.

Turning toward each other is one of the most important habits you can cultivate in a relationship. It's not about grand gestures, but about consistently showing up for your partner in the small moments that make up everyday life. By being present, responding with empathy, and showing affection, you can strengthen your emotional bond and build a relationship that is resilient, fulfilling, and full of love.

In the long run, turning toward each other creates a positive cycle of connection that helps couples navigate challenges, deepen intimacy, and maintain a strong emotional foundation. It's these everyday moments of turning toward each other that ultimately create the lasting closeness and happiness that every couple desires.

The Value of Emotional Support

In any healthy and lasting relationship, emotional support is one of the most important ingredients. It's not just about being there during life's big events or crises; emotional support is about showing up for your partner in the everyday moments, being a steady source of encouragement, comfort, and care. It's the foundation upon which trust, intimacy, and connection are built.

Emotional support means offering empathy when your partner is feeling down, celebrating their successes with genuine joy, and simply being a safe space where they can express themselves without fear of judgment. It strengthens the bond between partners, helping them feel understood, valued, and secure. While love might spark a relationship, it's emotional support that keeps it strong over the years.

Why Emotional Support Matters

The presence of emotional support in a relationship offers numerous benefits that can elevate both individual well-being and the overall health of the relationship. Here are some key reasons why emotional support is so valuable:

1. Fostering a Sense of Safety and Security

One of the primary roles of emotional support is to create a sense of safety within a relationship. When you know your partner is there for you emotionally, it builds a sense of trust and security that allows you to be vulnerable. Whether you're facing personal struggles or relationship challenges, knowing that your partner will support you through it fosters a deep sense of emotional safety. This is essential for building and maintaining a close, loving bond.

Emotional support acts as a safety net during stressful times. Life inevitably brings moments of difficulty—whether it's work stress, family issues, or personal challenges—but knowing that your partner has your back can help ease the burden. When you're emotionally supported, you're not just handling these challenges alone; you have a teammate who will walk with you through it all.

2. Enhancing Emotional Intimacy

Emotional intimacy is the closeness that develops when two people can share their innermost thoughts and feelings without fear of being judged or dismissed. Emotional support is what makes this intimacy possible. When partners are emotionally supportive of one another, they create a space where both feel comfortable sharing their joys, fears, frustrations, and dreams. This deepens the connection and allows for a more fulfilling and meaningful relationship.

By offering consistent emotional support, partners build a strong foundation of trust and openness. This level of emotional intimacy helps both people feel seen and heard, which is vital for maintaining a healthy, loving relationship.

3. Building Resilience Together

Relationships face challenges from time to time, whether it's an external stressor like financial troubles, health issues, or an internal struggle such as a disagreement or misunderstanding.

Emotional support helps couples weather these storms together. When partners provide emotional encouragement and reassurance to each other, they strengthen their resilience as a team.

With emotional support, couples are better able to navigate difficult situations without becoming disconnected or overwhelmed by stress. The act of supporting each other emotionally reinforces the idea that you're in it together, no matter what life throws your way.

4. Boosting Emotional Well-Being

Beyond strengthening the relationship, emotional support also has a profound impact on individual well-being. When you feel emotionally supported by your partner, it reduces feelings of loneliness, stress, and anxiety. It boosts self-esteem because it reminds you that you are valued and loved just as you are.

Supportive relationships contribute to better mental health, as people who feel emotionally connected to their partners tend to experience lower rates of depression and anxiety. Knowing that your partner cares for your emotional needs enhances your sense of self-worth and makes it easier to cope with life's challenges.

5. Deepening Communication

When emotional support is present, it fosters open and honest communication. Couples who feel emotionally safe with each other are more likely to express their true feelings and discuss important topics without fear of conflict or judgment. This leads to healthier, more transparent communication patterns and helps prevent misunderstandings from escalating into bigger issues.

Open communication fueled by emotional support also makes it easier to resolve conflicts in a constructive way. When partners know that they are supported, they are less likely to become defensive or shut down during difficult conversations. Instead, they are more willing to listen and collaborate on finding solutions that work for both parties.

How to Offer Emotional Support

Providing emotional support requires empathy, patience, and a willingness to be present for your partner, no matter the circumstances. Here are some practical ways to offer emotional support in your relationship:

1. Be a Good Listener

One of the most powerful forms of emotional support is simply listening. When your partner is expressing their thoughts or feelings, be fully present and give them your undivided attention. Avoid interrupting or offering solutions unless they specifically ask for advice. Instead, listen with empathy and validation. Let your partner know that their feelings matter and that you are there to understand them.

Sometimes, all a person needs is to be heard. By being a good listener, you provide a safe space for your partner to process their emotions and feel supported.

2. Show Empathy

Empathy is the ability to understand and share the feelings of another person. When your partner is going through a difficult time, offer empathy by acknowledging their emotions and validating their experience. Saying things like, "I can see why you're feeling that way" or "That sounds really hard" shows that you are tuned in to their emotional state.

Empathy is about being emotionally attuned to your partner's needs and making an effort to walk in their shoes. It's a powerful way to show that you care and that you're there for them no matter what.

3. Offer Encouragement and Reassurance

Sometimes, offering emotional support means being a source of encouragement and reassurance. If your partner is feeling unsure, anxious, or overwhelmed, let them know that you believe in them. Offer words of encouragement, reminding them of their strengths and abilities. Reassure them that, no matter what, you'll be by their side.

Even in small moments, offering a comforting word or a gesture of reassurance can make a big difference in how supported your partner feels.

4. Be There in Tough Times

Emotional support isn't just about showing up during the happy moments—it's about being there through the tough times as well. Whether your partner is dealing with personal challenges, work stress, or loss, your presence is invaluable.

Sometimes, just being there—whether it's holding their hand, giving them a hug, or sitting in silence with them—can provide immense comfort.

When your partner is struggling, your consistent presence sends a message that they are not alone in their hardship, and that you are a dependable source of support.

5. Celebrate Successes Together
Emotional support isn't only about offering comfort during difficult times. It also means celebrating your partner's successes and accomplishments. Whether it's a promotion at work, a personal achievement, or even a small win, take time to acknowledge and celebrate these moments together.

Sharing in each other's joy fosters a sense of partnership and strengthens the emotional bond between you. It shows that you are invested in your partner's happiness and growth.

The value of emotional support in a relationship cannot be overstated. It's the foundation of trust, intimacy, and resilience, allowing couples to feel secure, connected, and loved. Emotional support strengthens the bond between partners, providing a safe space for both to share their innermost thoughts and feelings.

By offering empathy, being a good listener, and consistently showing up for each other, couples can cultivate a deep emotional connection that carries them through both the good times and the difficult ones. Emotional support not only makes relationships stronger but also enhances the emotional well-being of both partners, creating a sense of security and partnership that can weather any storm.

Recognizing and Responding to Bids for Connection

In every relationship, there are countless moments when one partner reaches out to the other in small, often subtle ways. These moments are known as bids for connection—gestures, words, or actions that signal a desire for attention, affection, or support. Understanding how to recognize and respond to these bids is crucial for maintaining emotional intimacy and strengthening the bond between partners. It's these everyday interactions, more than grand romantic gestures, that build the foundation of a strong, loving relationship.

Bids for connection can be easy to miss if we're not paying attention. They can be as small as a smile, a casual comment, or a touch on the arm. But how we respond to these bids over time shapes the overall emotional climate of the relationship. Couples who consistently acknowledge and respond positively to each other's bids for connection are more likely to feel satisfied, close, and emotionally secure.

What Are Bids for Connection?

A bid for connection is any attempt by one partner to engage the other emotionally. It can be a direct request, like asking for help or advice, or something less obvious, like a playful nudge, sharing a random thought, or even making a joke. Bids are essentially efforts to establish or maintain emotional closeness.

Examples of bids for connection include:
- Asking a question: "How was your day?"
- Making an observation: "Look at that beautiful sunset."
- Offering physical affection: holding hands, a kiss, or a hug.
- Sharing something personal: "I've been feeling a little overwhelmed lately."
- Expressing a need: "Can we talk about something that's bothering me?"

These moments provide opportunities to connect on an emotional level. When one partner makes a bid, they are seeking acknowledgment, attention, or understanding from the other. How you respond to these bids can have a significant impact on the health and longevity of your relationship.

The Importance of Responding to Bids

When a bid for connection is made, you have three possible ways to respond: you can turn toward your partner, turn away, or turn against them. Each of these responses has a different effect on the relationship.

1. Turning Toward Your Partner

Turning toward your partner means acknowledging their bid in a positive, engaging way. It shows that you are interested in what they have to say or share, and that you value the connection. For example, if your partner says, "Look at that sunset," turning toward them might mean stopping what you're doing, looking at the sunset, and saying, "Wow, that's beautiful." It's a small act, but it makes your partner feel seen and appreciated.

Over time, turning toward your partner consistently creates a pattern of emotional closeness and trust. It strengthens the bond between you and fosters a sense of partnership. Research shows that couples who turn toward each other regularly are more likely to have successful, long-lasting relationships.

2. Turning Away from Your Partner

Turning away from your partner happens when you ignore or dismiss their bid for connection. This might look like being too absorbed in your phone to respond to their question, or simply brushing off a comment they make. When you turn away from a bid, it creates a small emotional disconnect. While this might not seem like a big deal in isolation, repeated instances of turning away can accumulate over time and create feelings of neglect or rejection.

In a relationship where bids are frequently ignored, one partner may eventually stop trying to connect altogether, leading to emotional distance and dissatisfaction.

3. Turning Against Your Partner

Turning against your partner means responding to their bid in a negative or hostile way. This can involve sarcasm, criticism, or irritation. For example, if your partner says, "Look at that sunset," and you respond with, "I'm busy. I don't have time for that right now," you're turning against them. These kinds of responses can damage the relationship, creating resentment and frustration.

When partners consistently turn against each other, it undermines trust and emotional security, making it difficult for the relationship to thrive.

Why Bids for Connection Matter

Bids for connection might seem small or insignificant in the moment, but over time, they form the backbone of a relationship's emotional health. Each bid is an opportunity to reinforce the emotional bond between partners. Consistently turning toward each other in these moments helps build a reservoir of positive feelings, which can make it easier to navigate challenges and disagreements when they arise.

Couples who frequently acknowledge and respond to each other's bids tend to feel more connected and satisfied in their relationships. On the other hand, relationships in which bids are often ignored or met with hostility are more likely to experience emotional distance, frustration, and even eventual breakdown.

How to Recognize Bids for Connection

Recognizing bids for connection requires being mindful and present in your interactions with your partner. Since bids can be subtle, it's easy to miss them, especially if you're distracted or preoccupied. Here are a few tips for recognizing your partner's bids:

1. Pay Attention to Nonverbal Cues

Bids for connection aren't always verbal. Sometimes they come in the form of body language, facial expressions, or physical gestures. For example, if your partner leans in for a hug or reaches out to hold your hand, that's a bid for connection. Being mindful of these nonverbal cues can help you respond in a way that fosters closeness.

2. Listen for Underlying Emotions

Sometimes a bid for connection is hidden beneath a seemingly mundane comment. If your partner says something like, "I'm exhausted," or "Work has been so stressful lately," they may be seeking emotional support or understanding. It's important to listen beyond the words and recognize when your partner is expressing a need for connection.

3. Be Present in the Moment

In today's busy world, it's easy to be distracted by work, technology, or other responsibilities. But being present in the moment with your partner is crucial for recognizing their bids for connection. Practice putting down your phone, turning off the TV, or stepping away from other distractions when your partner is talking to you. This allows you to be more attuned to their emotional needs and respond with care.

How to Respond to Bids for Connection

Once you recognize a bid, responding in a positive and supportive way can help strengthen your relationship. Here are some strategies for turning toward your partner's bids:

1. Acknowledge the Bid

Even if you're busy or distracted, acknowledging your partner's bid shows that you care. This could be as simple as making eye contact, offering a smile, or saying, "I hear you." The key is to show that you recognize their effort to connect with you.

2. Engage with Curiosity

If your partner makes a comment or asks a question, engage with curiosity. Ask follow-up questions, share your thoughts, or offer a response that shows genuine interest. For example, if your partner says, "I had such a stressful day at work," instead of brushing it off, you could ask, "What happened?" or "How are you feeling now?"

3. Show Empathy and Support

When your partner expresses a need or shares an emotion, offer empathy and support. This could be a comforting word, a reassuring touch, or simply listening without judgment. Let your partner know that you're there for them and that their feelings are valid.

4. Create Opportunities for Connection

Sometimes, turning toward your partner's bids can be as simple as creating opportunities for connection. Initiate a conversation, share something interesting or meaningful from your day, or suggest spending quality time together. These moments of connection help keep the emotional bond strong.

Recognizing and responding to bids for connection is one of the most important skills in a relationship. These everyday moments of emotional outreach are the building blocks of intimacy, trust, and love. By being present, attuned, and responsive, you can strengthen your relationship and create a deeper sense of emotional closeness.

Turning toward your partner's bids doesn't require grand gestures or major effort—it's about being there in the small moments, showing that you care, and making an intentional choice to connect. Over time, this consistent effort creates a strong, resilient relationship that can weather challenges and continue to grow in love and understanding.

Chapter 4: Allow Your Partner to Influence You

A key ingredient to a happy, lasting marriage is the ability to allow your partner to influence you. At first glance, the idea of being "influenced" might sound like losing control or making sacrifices, but it's not about one partner dominating the other. Instead, it's about mutual respect, collaboration, and openness to your partner's thoughts, opinions, and feelings. It's about embracing your partner as an equal, recognizing that both of you bring valuable perspectives and strengths to the relationship.

In relationships where partners allow each other to influence their decisions, there is less conflict and more shared decision-making. This practice creates a partnership in which both individuals feel valued and respected. It's not about one person getting their way all the time but about finding a balance where both partners contribute to the decisions that shape their lives together.

The Importance of Mutual Influence

At the heart of allowing your partner to influence you is the principle of mutual respect. When you consider your partner's feelings and input, you send the message that their opinions matter. This builds trust and emotional connection, which strengthens the overall foundation of the relationship. In contrast, when partners resist being influenced by each other—either by stubbornly holding onto their own views or dismissing the other's—it can lead to frustration, power struggles, and emotional distance.

Healthy relationships are dynamic, with both partners sharing power and responsibility. This give-and-take allows for more harmonious decision-making and a more satisfying partnership. When both individuals have a say, both feel heard and respected, which creates a sense of fairness and equality in the relationship.

1. Creating a Collaborative Relationship

When you allow your partner to influence you, you're actively engaging in collaboration. This means approaching your relationship as a team, rather than as two individuals who are constantly negotiating for control. It's about recognizing that, as partners, you are working together toward shared goals. Whether it's deciding where to live, how to raise your children, or what to have for dinner, making decisions collaboratively strengthens your connection.

When you collaborate, you show that you trust your partner's judgment and value their input. It also encourages more open communication because both partners feel safe in sharing their thoughts and opinions, knowing they will be taken seriously.

2. Avoiding Power Struggles

In many relationships, disagreements can turn into power struggles when one partner refuses to be influenced. This can happen when one person feels they always need to be right or maintain control. But in a healthy marriage, power is shared, not held tightly by one individual. When partners refuse to budge or consider each other's perspectives, it creates tension, resentment, and conflict.

Allowing your partner to influence you doesn't mean always giving in or letting go of your own opinions. Rather, it means being open to hearing their point of view and being willing to adjust your own stance when it makes sense. It's about flexibility and compromise, which helps avoid the tug-of-war that power struggles create.

3. Valuing Your Partner's Strengths

Every person brings unique strengths, experiences, and wisdom to a relationship. By allowing your partner to influence you, you are acknowledging and valuing their strengths. For example, if your partner is particularly good at managing finances, it makes sense to trust their judgment when it comes to financial decisions. Or, if your partner has a deep understanding of parenting strategies, being open to their insights can lead to better outcomes for your family.

Recognizing and appreciating your partner's strengths doesn't diminish your own abilities. Instead, it enhances the partnership because both individuals are contributing their best selves to the relationship. When you value each other's strengths, you create a more balanced and effective partnership.

How to Allow Your Partner to Influence You

Allowing influence doesn't come naturally to everyone, especially if you're used to being independent or if you've been raised in an environment that encouraged self-reliance over collaboration. But the good news is that this skill can be developed with intention and practice. Here are some ways to foster a relationship where both partners can influence each other positively:

1. Listen with an Open Mind

The first step in allowing your partner to influence you is being a good listener. When your partner expresses their thoughts, opinions, or desires, listen without judgment or defensiveness. Try to understand where they are coming from and why they feel the way they do. Active listening requires more than just hearing the words—it means truly trying to understand your partner's perspective.

An open mind means you're willing to consider the possibility that your partner's idea may be as good or better than your own. It's about letting go of the need to be right and embracing the idea that your partner's input is valuable.

2. Be Willing to Compromise

Healthy relationships are built on compromise. This doesn't mean you have to give up on your own needs or desires, but it does mean being flexible and finding solutions that work for both of you. Compromise is the cornerstone of shared decision-making.

For example, if you and your partner are deciding on a vacation destination and you both have different preferences, instead of one person insisting on their choice, look for a compromise. Maybe you can alternate vacation spots or choose a destination that incorporates elements of both of your preferences. The goal is to reach a decision that makes both partners feel satisfied.

3. Respect Your Partner's Feelings and Opinions

Even when you disagree with your partner, it's important to respect their feelings and opinions. Dismissing or belittling your partner's perspective can damage the trust and respect that are essential to a healthy relationship. Instead, approach disagreements with kindness and a willingness to understand.

Respecting your partner's opinions doesn't mean you always have to agree, but it does mean acknowledging that their perspective is valid. By showing respect, you create a safe environment where both partners feel comfortable expressing themselves.

4. Express Your Own Needs Clearly

Allowing your partner to influence you doesn't mean silencing your own voice. It's important to express your own needs, desires, and opinions in a clear and respectful way. A relationship where only one partner's voice is heard isn't truly collaborative. When both partners are able to express themselves, it leads to healthier, more balanced decision-making.

Being assertive about your needs while remaining open to your partner's influence is key to maintaining a healthy balance in the relationship. It's not about one person always deferring to the other—it's about creating a dialogue where both partners contribute equally.

5. Recognize When to Let Go

In some situations, it's important to recognize when to let go of your own position and allow your partner to take the lead. This doesn't mean giving in every time, but rather understanding that in certain areas, your partner's perspective might be more informed or beneficial.

For example, if your partner is more knowledgeable about a particular subject—whether it's home improvement, finances, or planning social events—trusting their judgment can lead to better outcomes for both of you. Letting go of control in these situations shows trust and respect for your partner's expertise.

The Benefits of Allowing Influence

Allowing your partner to influence you leads to a more harmonious, respectful, and emotionally connected relationship. When both partners feel heard, valued, and respected, it deepens the emotional bond between them. Here are some key benefits of allowing influence:

1. Stronger Emotional Connection

When partners allow each other to influence their decisions, it creates a sense of partnership and teamwork. This leads to a stronger emotional connection, as both individuals feel valued and supported.

2. Reduced Conflict

When couples share power and decision-making, there's less room for conflict. Instead of engaging in power struggles, partners collaborate to find solutions that work for both of them, reducing tension and resentment.

3. Increased Trust

Allowing your partner to influence you builds trust. It shows that you respect their opinions and trust their judgment. Over time, this trust deepens, making the relationship more secure and stable.

4. Mutual Growth

By being open to your partner's influence, you allow room for growth—both individually and as a couple. You learn from each other's perspectives and experiences, which enriches the relationship and helps both partners grow.

Allowing your partner to influence you is an essential part of building a strong, lasting relationship. It's not about giving up control or being passive—it's about embracing your partner as an equal and creating a collaborative, respectful partnership. By listening with an open mind, being willing to compromise, and respecting each other's opinions, you can build a relationship based on trust, emotional connection, and shared decision-making.

When both partners feel valued and heard, the relationship thrives. Allowing influence is a sign of mutual respect, and it strengthens the bond that keeps couples together through the ups and downs of life.

Embracing Mutual Respect and Compromise

Mutual respect and compromise are two cornerstones of a successful and healthy marriage. They act as the glue that holds a relationship together, fostering an environment where both partners feel valued, heard, and supported. While love may spark a relationship, mutual respect and compromise help it grow and flourish, even through difficult times.

Understanding and embracing these principles doesn't just help resolve conflicts—it strengthens the bond between partners, creates a sense of equality, and promotes a lasting emotional connection. In this chapter, we'll dive deep into what mutual respect and compromise look like in a marriage and how you can cultivate them in your relationship.

What is Mutual Respect?

At its core, mutual respect is about valuing your partner as an individual, acknowledging their worth, and treating them with kindness and consideration. Respect in a marriage means appreciating your partner's unique qualities, supporting their dreams, and recognizing that their needs and opinions are just as important as your own.

In a respectful relationship, partners listen to each other, even when they disagree. They engage in open communication, refrain from dismissive or demeaning behavior, and work together as equals. Mutual respect is the foundation for trust and emotional safety in a relationship.

The Importance of Respect

Without respect, love alone is not enough to sustain a marriage. Couples who don't respect each other often find themselves stuck in cycles of conflict, frustration, and emotional distance. Respect prevents the kind of hurtful behaviors that erode trust—like criticism, contempt, and dismissiveness. When partners respect each other, they create a safe space where both individuals can express themselves freely without fear of judgment or rejection.

In addition, respect fosters a deeper emotional connection. When you show respect to your partner, you acknowledge their humanity, their individuality, and their needs. This creates a sense of belonging and security, knowing that you're in a relationship where both partners are valued.

What Does Respect Look Like in a Marriage?

Respect in a marriage can manifest in many ways, from how you communicate with each other to how you navigate differences. Here are some key behaviors that demonstrate respect in a relationship:

1. Active Listening

One of the simplest and most effective ways to show respect is by truly listening to your partner. This means giving them your full attention, making eye contact, and engaging with what they're saying, rather than just waiting for your turn to speak.

Active listening shows your partner that their thoughts and feelings matter to you.

2. Valuing Each Other's Opinions

In any marriage, there will be times when you and your partner don't see eye to eye. However, respect means acknowledging that your partner's opinions are just as valid as your own, even if you disagree. Instead of dismissing or belittling their perspective, try to understand where they're coming from.

3. Avoiding Harmful Criticism

Disagreements are inevitable in any relationship, but how you handle them can make a big difference. Respectful partners avoid using harmful criticism or personal attacks. Instead of saying, "You're always so lazy," a respectful approach would be, "I feel overwhelmed when there's a lot to do around the house. Can we work on finding a better system together?"

4. Supporting Each Other's Growth

Respect also means supporting your partner's personal growth and aspirations. This involves being their cheerleader in both big and small ways, encouraging them to pursue their goals, and celebrating their successes. A marriage built on respect is one where both partners feel empowered to grow, both individually and as a couple.

5. Setting and Honoring Boundaries

Every individual has personal boundaries—whether emotional, physical, or mental. Respecting these boundaries is crucial for a healthy marriage. This means not pushing your partner to do things they're uncomfortable with and being mindful of their limits. Honoring boundaries creates a safe and trusting environment in the relationship.

The Role of Compromise in Marriage

Compromise is another essential element of a strong marriage. At its heart, compromise is about finding a middle ground where both partners can feel satisfied. It's not about one person always getting their way or one partner making all the sacrifices—it's about creating solutions that work for both people in the relationship.

Marriage involves two individuals with different experiences, opinions, and preferences, and compromise helps bridge those differences. Whether it's deciding how to spend money, how to parent children, or even what to watch on TV, compromise is an ongoing process of negotiation and balance.

Why Compromise Matters

Compromise shows that you're willing to put the needs of the relationship above your own ego or desire to "win" an argument. It demonstrates that you value your partner's happiness as much as your own and that you're committed to finding solutions that work for both of you.

When compromise is absent in a marriage, one or both partners may feel resentful or unheard. Over time, this can lead to feelings of imbalance or dissatisfaction. On the other hand, couples who practice compromise regularly build trust and cooperation, which strengthens their bond and helps prevent conflicts from escalating.

How to Compromise Effectively

Compromise requires patience, empathy, and open communication. Here are some strategies to help you and your partner navigate compromise in a healthy way:

1. Be Open to Dialogue

Healthy compromise starts with communication. Instead of assuming you know what your partner wants, engage in a conversation where both of you can express your needs and concerns. By clearly communicating your desires, you'll be better equipped to find solutions that work for both of you.

2. Focus on the Big Picture

Sometimes, letting go of small preferences in favor of your partner's needs can lead to greater harmony in the relationship. Ask yourself whether this issue is worth holding onto or whether it's something you can let go of for the sake of peace and connection. Focusing on the bigger picture—your overall happiness and the health of the relationship—can help you determine when compromise is worth it.

3. Find a Middle Ground

Compromise doesn't mean one person always gives in; it means finding a middle ground where both partners feel satisfied. This may involve creative problem-solving or combining both partners' ideas. For example, if one partner wants to save money while the other wants a vacation, the compromise might be a more affordable getaway that still offers relaxation without breaking the bank.

4. Avoid Keeping Score

In a healthy marriage, compromise isn't about keeping track of who has given up more or who "owes" the other person. Instead, it's about creating balance and fairness. When partners start keeping score, it can lead to resentment and competitiveness, which erode the spirit of collaboration. Instead, approach each situation with the goal of maintaining harmony, not winning points.

5. Respect Differences

Compromise doesn't mean you have to agree on everything. It's perfectly okay to have different preferences, as long as you can find ways to respect those differences and find common ground. Recognize that differences can add richness to the relationship rather than being sources of conflict.

The Balance Between Respect and Compromise

Respect and compromise go hand in hand in a healthy marriage. Without respect, compromise can feel forced or insincere. And without compromise, respect may not translate into meaningful action. Together, these principles create a partnership that thrives on mutual understanding and cooperation.

When you respect your partner, you're more likely to engage in healthy compromise because you value their needs and feelings. Likewise, when you compromise, you're showing respect by acknowledging that both partners' needs are important.

Mutual respect and compromise are the building blocks of a strong, fulfilling marriage. They help couples navigate the challenges of life together, fostering a relationship based on trust, equality, and shared responsibility. By respecting each other's individuality and working together to find common ground, partners create a deep, lasting bond that can withstand the test of time.

Embracing these principles is not always easy—it requires patience, understanding, and a willingness to put the relationship first. But the rewards are immense. A marriage built on respect and compromise is one where both partners feel loved, supported, and truly seen for who they are.

Making Decisions Together

In a healthy and thriving marriage, making decisions together is one of the most important aspects of maintaining a balanced and supportive relationship. It's about more than simply splitting responsibilities—it's about fostering a sense of partnership and equality where both partners feel empowered, respected, and heard. Collaborative decision-making strengthens the bond between spouses and helps create an atmosphere of mutual respect and trust.

The Power of Shared Decision-Making

Marriage is a partnership, and in a partnership, decisions affect both people. Whether it's a big decision, like buying a house, or smaller daily choices, such as what to cook for dinner, involving both partners in the decision-making process ensures that each person's opinions and feelings are considered. When decisions are made together, both partners feel a sense of ownership and responsibility for the outcome, which helps to foster cooperation and avoid potential resentment.

Shared decision-making isn't about one person "winning" or "losing" in a discussion—it's about finding a solution that works for both partners. This means considering each other's perspectives, weighing options together, and working toward a common goal.

Why It's Important to Make Decisions Together
When couples make decisions together, it reflects a fundamental level of respect and care in the relationship. Here are a few reasons why this practice is so important:

1. It Strengthens Emotional Bonds
When partners collaborate on decisions, it reinforces the emotional connection between them. The act of discussing, debating, and deciding together is a form of intimacy—it shows that you're not just two individuals with separate lives, but a team that faces challenges and opportunities together. This sense of unity deepens trust and strengthens the bond between you and your spouse.

2. It Creates a Sense of Equality

In a balanced and healthy marriage, both partners have an equal voice in decisions that affect their lives. When only one person consistently makes the decisions, the relationship can start to feel unequal, with one person exerting control and the other feeling sidelined or powerless. Making decisions together creates a sense of equality and fairness, where both partners' opinions are respected and valued.

3. It Prevents Resentment

When one person consistently makes decisions without consulting their partner, it can lead to feelings of frustration and resentment. Over time, this can cause emotional distance, as one partner feels like their opinions aren't valued. Making decisions together helps prevent these feelings from building up by ensuring that both partners are involved and invested in the outcomes.

4. It Promotes Better Problem-Solving

Two heads are better than one. When couples make decisions together, they can draw from each other's strengths, experiences, and perspectives. This often leads to better solutions than if one person made the decision on their own. Shared decision-making allows for a more well-rounded view of a situation and ensures that the couple is working together to solve problems effectively.

How to Make Decisions Together

While making decisions together sounds simple, it can sometimes be challenging, especially when partners have different viewpoints or preferences. Here are some strategies to help couples navigate decision-making in a collaborative and respectful way:

1. Communicate Openly and Honestly

Clear and honest communication is the foundation of making decisions together. When faced with a decision, it's important for both partners to share their thoughts, feelings, and concerns. Avoid assuming that your partner knows what you're thinking—express your desires and preferences openly.

During discussions, listen actively to what your partner has to say. This means not just hearing their words, but understanding their point of view. When both partners feel heard and understood, it becomes easier to find common ground and make decisions together.

2. Be Willing to Compromise

Compromise is an essential part of decision-making in any relationship. There will be times when you and your partner have different opinions, and in these moments, it's important to find a middle ground that works for both of you. Compromise doesn't mean sacrificing your needs or giving in to your partner's desires every time—it's about finding a solution that honors both of your perspectives.

In some cases, it may be helpful to prioritize different decisions. For example, if one partner feels strongly about a particular issue, the other partner might be willing to compromise more on that decision, knowing that their preferences will be prioritized in another area.

3. Respect Each Other's Expertise

In many relationships, each partner brings different strengths and areas of expertise to the table. Recognizing and respecting these strengths can help with decision-making. For example, if one partner is more knowledgeable about finances, it may make sense to lean on their expertise when making financial decisions. Similarly, if one partner has a deeper understanding of home improvement, their input might carry more weight when making decisions about home repairs or renovations.

Respecting each other's expertise doesn't mean one person gets to make all the decisions in a particular area—it means valuing each other's strengths and using them to enhance the decision-making process.

4. Take Your Time

Rushed decisions often lead to regret or conflict later on. If a decision doesn't need to be made immediately, take the time to discuss it thoroughly with your partner. Allowing space for reflection can help both of you feel more confident in the choice you make together. Taking the time to weigh all options carefully ensures that both partners are fully on board with the final decision.

5. Avoid Power Struggles

In some relationships, decision-making can become a battleground where one partner tries to assert control over the other. This leads to power struggles, which can cause tension and resentment. To avoid this, focus on working as a team rather than competing to "win" the argument. Remember that you're both working toward the same goal—making the best decision for your relationship.

6. Use the "We" Approach

A helpful way to frame decision-making is to think of it as a "we" process rather than a "me" or "you" process. Using language like "What should we do?" or "How can we make this work for both of us?" reinforces the idea that decisions are made together, as a team. This mindset helps shift the focus away from individual desires and onto shared goals.

Making Major vs. Minor Decisions

Not all decisions carry the same weight in a marriage. Some decisions—such as where to live, whether to have children, or how to manage finances—require deep discussion and careful consideration. Other decisions—like what to have for dinner or which movie to watch—are more minor and can often be handled quickly or with less intensity.

For minor decisions, it's important to pick your battles and not get bogged down in every small detail. In many cases, it's perfectly fine to let your partner take the lead or to alternate decision-making on smaller issues. For major decisions, though, it's crucial that both partners are involved and fully invested in the process.

The Benefits of Making Decisions Together
When couples make decisions together, the benefits ripple throughout the relationship:

1. Increased Trust
Shared decision-making builds trust because both partners feel that their opinions are valued. Trust grows when couples know they can rely on each other to collaborate and support each other's needs.

2. Stronger Partnership
Working together to make decisions strengthens the partnership and reinforces the idea that you're both in this together. This sense of teamwork can help couples navigate the challenges of life with greater resilience.

3. Reduced Conflict
When decisions are made unilaterally, it can lead to frustration and conflict. In contrast, making decisions together reduces the likelihood of misunderstandings and disagreements, as both partners have been part of the process from the beginning.

4. Greater Satisfaction
Couples who make decisions together tend to feel more satisfied in their relationship because both partners are involved in shaping the direction of their lives. When decisions are made collaboratively, there's a greater sense of fulfillment and happiness in the relationship.

Making decisions together is a vital aspect of a healthy marriage. It reinforces the bond between partners, promotes equality, and helps prevent resentment or conflict. By communicating openly, compromising when necessary, and respecting each other's input, couples can make decisions that are not only practical but also strengthen their emotional connection.

In the end, decision-making isn't just about resolving specific issues—it's about creating a collaborative, respectful partnership where both partners feel heard, valued, and supported. Through shared decision-making, couples can build a relationship that is stronger, more resilient, and deeply fulfilling.

Chapter 5: Solving Your Solvable Problems

Every marriage will face challenges—some big, some small. But not all problems are created equal. Some conflicts are perpetual, stemming from fundamental differences in personality or values, while others are solvable—issues that can be resolved through communication, understanding, and compromise. In this chapter, we focus on how to effectively address and solve the solvable problems in your marriage.

When couples learn to identify which problems can be solved and approach them with the right strategies, they can greatly reduce the stress and tension that can accumulate over time. Addressing solvable problems also strengthens the bond between partners by reinforcing teamwork and fostering a sense of accomplishment. So, what's the key to solving problems? A combination of clear communication, mutual respect, and a willingness to compromise.

Understanding Solvable vs. Perpetual Problems

Before diving into strategies for solving problems, it's important to distinguish between solvable and perpetual problems. Solvable problems are those that have a clear solution, often involving temporary issues such as household chores, financial decisions, or social activities. These are the types of problems that, with effort and communication, can be resolved to the satisfaction of both partners.

On the other hand, perpetual problems stem from deeper, ongoing differences in personality, values, or life goals. These might include differing desires about having children, differences in spending habits, or contrasting lifestyles. Perpetual problems require long-term strategies for managing them rather than solving them entirely, as they often reflect fundamental differences in how partners see the world.

Focusing on solvable problems is crucial because it gives couples a sense of progress and accomplishment. Tackling these issues helps reduce day-to-day frustrations and opens up more space for emotional intimacy and connection.

Step-by-Step Process for Solving Problems
When you approach a solvable problem in your marriage, it's important to use a structured and respectful process to work through it. Let's walk through the key steps for resolving issues effectively:

1. Identify the Problem Clearly
The first step in solving any problem is to identify it clearly. Often, couples get stuck because they argue about symptoms of a problem without addressing the root cause. For example, frequent arguments about who does the dishes might reflect a deeper issue of feeling unappreciated or overwhelmed by household responsibilities.

To identify the problem, ask yourselves:
- What exactly are we arguing about?
- What specific behavior or situation is causing tension?
- Are there underlying emotional needs or concerns contributing to the problem?

Once you've pinpointed the issue, you can move forward with finding a solution that addresses the heart of the matter, rather than just its surface symptoms.

2. Approach the Problem with a Positive Mindset

How you approach a problem has a huge impact on how successfully you'll solve it. If you approach the issue with criticism, blame, or defensiveness, it's likely to escalate into a bigger conflict. Instead, try to approach the problem with a positive and cooperative mindset.

One way to do this is by focusing on the solution rather than the fault. For example, instead of saying, "You never help around the house," try framing it as, "I've been feeling overwhelmed with the housework lately. Can we find a way to split the chores more evenly?"

This shift in tone shows that you're interested in finding a solution rather than attacking your partner. It also encourages cooperation, as your partner won't feel as if they need to defend themselves.

3. Practice Active Listening

Effective problem-solving in marriage requires both partners to listen to each other with empathy and understanding. This means truly hearing what your partner has to say without interrupting, dismissing, or jumping to conclusions.

Active listening involves:
- Giving your partner your full attention: Put aside distractions, make eye contact, and show through your body language that you're fully engaged in the conversation.
- Reflecting back what you've heard: After your partner has spoken, summarize what you've understood, such as, "It sounds like you're feeling stressed because you don't feel supported with the chores. Is that right?"
- Validating their feelings: Even if you don't agree with everything your partner says, acknowledge their feelings as valid. You might say, "I understand that you've been feeling overwhelmed, and I don't want you to feel that way."

By practicing active listening, both partners will feel heard and understood, which reduces defensiveness and opens the door to effective problem-solving.

4. Brainstorm Solutions Together

Once both partners have had a chance to express their thoughts and feelings, the next step is to brainstorm solutions together. Keep in mind that there's rarely only one "right" solution to a problem. Instead, aim for a solution that works for both partners, even if it requires compromise.

For example, if the problem is about household chores, you might brainstorm a variety of solutions:

Create a chore schedule where responsibilities are divided more evenly.
Hire outside help for specific tasks, if it's within your budget.
Set aside a specific time each week to tackle chores together.
As you brainstorm, focus on generating a variety of options without immediately dismissing any of them. The goal is to explore possibilities and find common ground.

5. Compromise Where Necessary

Compromise is often the key to solving solvable problems. In any marriage, there will be times when one or both partners need to make concessions to reach an agreement. Compromise doesn't mean giving in or sacrificing your needs—it means finding a middle ground where both partners can feel satisfied with the solution.

For example, if one partner prefers to spend weekends relaxing while the other prefers to tackle household projects, a compromise might involve setting aside Saturday mornings for chores and the rest of the weekend for relaxation.

The most important aspect of compromise is that both partners feel that their needs have been considered and that the solution is fair. If one person feels like they're always the one giving in, it can lead to resentment, so aim for balance in how compromises are made.

6. Follow Up and Adjust if Necessary

Once you've reached a solution and implemented it, it's important to follow up and check in with each other. Is the solution working? Are there any adjustments that need to be made? Following up ensures that the problem doesn't resurface and helps keep communication open.

If something isn't working, don't be afraid to revisit the issue and tweak your approach. Problem-solving is an ongoing process, and sometimes it takes a few tries to find a solution that sticks.

Common Solvable Problems in Marriage

There are many solvable problems that couples face throughout their marriage. Here are some common ones and potential strategies for solving them:

1. Division of Household Responsibilities

One of the most common sources of conflict in marriages is how to divide household chores. Couples can solve this problem by clearly communicating their expectations, creating a fair and balanced schedule, and being flexible as life circumstances change.

2. Financial Decisions

Money is often a source of tension in relationships, but it's also a solvable problem. Couples can address financial disagreements by setting a budget together, discussing long-term goals, and agreeing on how to manage joint and individual finances.

3. Parenting Styles

Differences in parenting approaches can cause friction, but they can also be addressed through open communication and compromise. Couples should discuss their values and priorities as parents and work together to find a parenting style that reflects both of their beliefs.

4. Social Activities and Hobbies

Couples may have different preferences when it comes to how they spend their free time. Solvable problems in this area can be addressed by balancing time spent together and apart, as well as finding activities that both partners enjoy.

Solving solvable problems is an essential skill for any married couple. By approaching issues with a positive mindset, practicing active listening, and being willing to compromise, couples can address conflicts in a way that strengthens their relationship and fosters greater intimacy. Remember, not every problem can be solved, but learning to handle the ones that can makes a huge difference in the overall health and happiness of your marriage.

Constructive Conflict Resolution Techniques

Conflict is a natural part of any marriage, and how couples navigate these disagreements significantly impacts their relationship's health. While arguments can create tension, they can also lead to deeper understanding and stronger connections when handled constructively. This chapter explores practical techniques for resolving conflicts that can help couples turn disagreements into opportunities for growth.

Understanding Conflict

Before diving into resolution techniques, it's important to recognize that conflict arises from differences in values, beliefs, and perspectives. Whether stemming from external stressors like work or family pressures, or internal issues such as communication styles, conflict is unavoidable. However, it's not the presence of conflict that determines a successful relationship but rather how partners choose to handle it. Constructive conflict resolution can lead to improved communication, increased intimacy, and a stronger partnership.

1. Create a Safe Space for Discussion

To resolve conflicts effectively, couples must first create an environment where both partners feel safe to express their feelings. This involves establishing ground rules for discussions, such as avoiding insults and staying focused on the issue at hand. Choosing a neutral and comfortable setting for conversations can help both partners feel more relaxed and open.

2. Use "I" Statements

One of the most effective communication techniques during a conflict is using **"I"** statements instead of **"you"** statements. This approach focuses on expressing one's own feelings rather than blaming the partner. For example, instead of saying, "You always ignore my needs," try expressing, "I feel neglected when my needs aren't considered." This small shift can reduce defensiveness and encourage a more open and honest dialogue.

3. Practice Active Listening

Active listening is crucial for understanding your partner's perspective. It involves giving full attention to your partner, acknowledging their feelings, and reflecting on what they say. To practice active listening:

- Maintain eye contact and nod to show engagement.
- Avoid interrupting or formulating your response while they speak.
- Summarize or paraphrase their points to confirm understanding, such as, "So what I'm hearing is that you feel…"

By demonstrating that you value your partner's perspective, you create a supportive atmosphere conducive to resolution.

4. Stay Focused on the Issue

During a conflict, it can be tempting to bring up past grievances or unrelated issues. However, staying focused on the current disagreement helps prevent escalation and confusion. If past conflicts arise, acknowledge them, but prioritize resolving the current issue first. Keeping the conversation centered on the matter at hand allows for a clearer and more effective resolution process.

5. Identify Underlying Needs

Many conflicts stem from unmet needs or emotional triggers. Understanding these underlying factors can help both partners find common ground. Encourage open dialogue about what each partner needs in the situation:

What do I feel I need right now?
What emotions are influencing my reactions?
By identifying these needs, couples can work together to address the root causes of the conflict, rather than just the symptoms.

6. Brainstorm Solutions Together

Once both partners have shared their feelings and needs, it's time to brainstorm potential solutions collaboratively. Encourage each other to suggest solutions, regardless of how practical they may seem. Discuss the pros and cons of each option and work together to create a resolution that respects both partners' needs. This collaborative approach fosters a sense of teamwork and reinforces the idea that both partners are committed to finding a mutually satisfactory outcome.

7. Take Breaks When Needed

If emotions escalate during a disagreement, it may be helpful to take a break. Stepping away from the conversation allows both partners to cool down and reflect on their feelings. During this time, it's important to agree on a specific timeframe to revisit the discussion, ensuring that the issue remains a priority. A timeout can prevent harmful exchanges and promote a more constructive dialogue when you reconvene.

8. Use Humor Wisely

A little humor can go a long way in diffusing tension during a conflict. Light-hearted jokes or playful banter can help remind both partners that they are on the same team. However, it's crucial to be sensitive and ensure that humor is appropriate and not dismissive of the issue at hand. When used wisely, humor can foster connection and ease the emotional intensity of a disagreement.

9. Seek to Understand Rather than to Win

The goal of constructive conflict resolution is not to "win" the argument but to understand each other better and find a solution that satisfies both partners. Approach conflicts with the mindset that you are allies working together to solve a problem. This perspective helps to build empathy and reinforces the importance of respect within the relationship.

10. Know When to Seek Professional Help

While many conflicts can be resolved with constructive techniques, some issues may require the assistance of a qualified therapist or counselor. If conflicts become frequent, intense, or feel insurmountable, seeking professional help can provide valuable tools and strategies for navigating conflicts more effectively. A neutral third party can offer insights that help couples communicate and resolve issues more constructively.

Constructive conflict resolution is an essential skill for maintaining a healthy and thriving marriage. By implementing these techniques—creating a safe environment, using "I" statements, practicing active listening, focusing on the issue, identifying needs, brainstorming solutions, taking breaks, using humor wisely, seeking understanding, and knowing when to seek help—couples can transform conflicts into opportunities for deeper connection and growth. Remember, it's not about avoiding conflict altogether but rather handling it in a way that strengthens your relationship and fosters mutual respect and understanding. With commitment and practice, couples can develop the skills necessary to navigate conflicts constructively, ultimately enhancing their bond and relationship satisfaction.

Approaches to Dealing With Everyday Disagreements
Every marriage experiences its fair share of disagreements, and navigating these differences is essential for a healthy, thriving relationship. While some conflicts are significant and require thoughtful resolution, many everyday disagreements can be addressed with simple strategies that promote understanding and cooperation. This chapter explores practical approaches to handling common disagreements in a way that fosters harmony and connection.

Acknowledge That Disagreements Are Normal

The first step in addressing everyday disagreements is to recognize that they are a normal part of any relationship. Every couple has different preferences, values, and perspectives, and these differences can lead to conflicts. Instead of viewing disagreements as a threat to the relationship, see them as opportunities for growth and understanding. Acknowledging that it's okay to disagree allows couples to approach conflicts with a more positive and open mindset.

1. Choose the Right Time and Place

When a disagreement arises, the timing and environment in which you discuss it can significantly impact the outcome. Avoid bringing up sensitive topics during stressful times or when either partner is preoccupied or tired. Instead, choose a time when both partners can engage in a calm and focused discussion. A quiet, private space can create a safe environment for open dialogue, allowing both partners to express their thoughts and feelings without distractions.

2. Practice Empathy and Understanding

During disagreements, it's crucial to approach your partner's perspective with empathy. Instead of immediately defending your viewpoint, take the time to understand where your partner is coming from. Ask open-ended questions and listen actively to their concerns. For example:

- "Can you help me understand why this is important to you?"
- "What do you feel about the situation?"

Practicing empathy helps create a more respectful dialogue and fosters a deeper emotional connection. When both partners feel heard and understood, it becomes easier to find common ground.

3. Keep Communication Open and Respectful

Clear, respectful communication is essential for resolving disagreements. Avoid using accusatory language or making sweeping generalizations, which can escalate tensions. Instead, focus on expressing your own feelings and opinions using "I" statements. For example, instead of saying, "You never listen to me," try saying, "I feel unheard when we discuss important matters." This approach encourages your partner to be more receptive to your perspective and less defensive.

Additionally, make an effort to maintain a calm tone and body language throughout the conversation. Nonverbal cues, such as eye contact and open posture, can convey respect and understanding, even during heated discussions.

4. Find Common Ground

In many disagreements, there is often a shared interest or common ground that both partners can agree on. Focus on identifying those areas of agreement as a starting point for resolution. For instance, if there's a disagreement about how to spend the weekend, you might both agree on the importance of quality time together. From there, you can explore different activities that align with that shared value.

By finding common ground, couples can create a collaborative atmosphere where both partners feel invested in reaching a mutually satisfying solution.

5. Be Willing to Compromise

Compromise is a vital skill in any relationship, especially when it comes to everyday disagreements. Sometimes, finding a solution requires both partners to adjust their expectations or make concessions. Approach compromise with an open mind, and be willing to discuss what each partner is willing to give and take.

For example, if one partner prefers a quiet night in while the other wants to go out with friends, a compromise might involve alternating between the two preferences. This way, both partners feel valued and respected, and it reinforces the idea that each partner's needs are important.

6. Take a Timeout if Needed

If tensions rise during a disagreement, it can be helpful to take a timeout. Stepping away for a short period allows both partners to cool down and reflect on their feelings without escalating the conflict further. Agree on a specific timeframe for reconvening the conversation, ensuring that the issue remains a priority for resolution.

During the timeout, each partner can engage in self-reflection, practicing mindfulness, or even discussing their feelings with a trusted friend or family member. This break can lead to more constructive conversations when you come back together.

7. Seek Solutions Together

Once both partners have shared their perspectives and emotions, the next step is to collaboratively brainstorm solutions. This process should focus on finding resolutions that satisfy both partners' needs. Encourage open dialogue about potential solutions, and don't be afraid to think outside the box.

Consider asking questions like:
- "What do you think would be a fair solution?"
- "How can we both feel comfortable with the outcome?"

By working together to find solutions, couples not only resolve the disagreement but also strengthen their partnership through teamwork.

8. Know When to Agree to Disagree

Not all disagreements will reach a resolution, and that's perfectly okay. Sometimes, couples may have differing opinions on issues that are deeply rooted in personal values or beliefs. In these situations, it's essential to recognize when to agree to disagree. This approach allows both partners to maintain their individuality while respecting each other's perspectives.

When agreeing to disagree, ensure that both partners acknowledge and validate each other's feelings. This acknowledgment reinforces the idea that differing viewpoints do not diminish the love and respect within the relationship.

Everyday disagreements are an inevitable part of married life, but how couples approach and manage these conflicts can make all the difference. By employing strategies such as empathy, respectful communication, compromise, and collaborative problem-solving, partners can navigate disagreements in a way that strengthens their relationship rather than weakens it. Remember, it's not about avoiding conflict but about handling it constructively, ensuring that both partners feel heard, valued, and understood. With these approaches, couples can turn everyday disagreements into opportunities for deeper connection and understanding, ultimately fostering a more harmonious and fulfilling marriage.

Chapter 6: Overcoming Conflict Gridlock

In any marriage, conflicts are bound to arise, and while some disagreements can be resolved easily, others can become stuck in what is often referred to as "gridlock." This term describes a situation where partners feel unable to move forward, leading to frustration, resentment, and a sense of hopelessness. Gridlock occurs when couples find themselves caught in a recurring cycle of disagreement, often on issues that are deeply rooted in personal values, beliefs, or life dreams. Understanding how to overcome this gridlock is essential for maintaining a healthy and fulfilling relationship.

Recognizing the Signs of Conflict Gridlock

The first step in overcoming conflict gridlock is recognizing its signs. Couples in gridlock may experience:

- Repeated Arguments: Constantly returning to the same issue without resolution.
- Resentment: Holding onto past grievances and allowing them to affect the current relationship.
- Withdrawal: Avoiding discussions about the issue altogether or feeling emotionally distant.

- Emotional Baggage: Allowing past conflicts to influence current interactions, leading to a lack of trust.

If you find yourself in this situation, it's crucial to address the gridlock before it begins to erode the foundation of your marriage.

Understanding the Underlying Issues

Often, gridlock is not merely about the surface issue at hand, such as household chores or financial decisions. Instead, these conflicts usually stem from deeper underlying needs or values. To effectively address gridlock, both partners must take the time to explore the root causes of their disagreements.

Consider these questions:

- What is at stake for each partner? Understanding what each person values can reveal the underlying fears and desires that fuel the conflict.
- What needs are not being met? This could include emotional needs for connection, respect, or security.
- How do past experiences shape your current perspectives? Reflecting on how individual backgrounds influence your responses can shed light on why certain issues are so contentious.

1. Approach the Issue with Curiosity

When tackling gridlocked issues, it's essential to approach the conversation with a sense of curiosity rather than judgment. Instead of trying to "fix" the problem immediately, focus on understanding each other's viewpoints. This means asking open-ended questions and genuinely listening to your partner's thoughts and feelings.

For example:
- "Can you help me understand why this issue is so important to you?"
- "What emotions come up for you when we discuss this topic?"

This inquisitive mindset encourages both partners to share their perspectives without feeling attacked or dismissed.

2. Identify Shared Goals

Another effective strategy for overcoming gridlock is to identify shared goals. Even in the midst of conflict, couples usually have common desires, such as wanting a harmonious home life or ensuring a happy, fulfilling relationship. By focusing on these shared goals, couples can work collaboratively to find a resolution that respects both partners' needs.

For instance, if the disagreement revolves around differing financial priorities, identify the shared goal of financial security. This common interest can help guide the conversation and promote a more cooperative atmosphere.

3. Explore Compromises and Alternatives

While some issues may seem insurmountable, there are often ways to explore compromises or alternative solutions. Once both partners understand each other's perspectives and shared goals, it's time to brainstorm possible compromises that respect both parties.

Consider these strategies:
- ***Creative Solutions:*** Encourage out-of-the-box thinking. Sometimes, a unique solution can satisfy both partners' needs.
- ***Trial Periods:*** Suggest implementing a temporary solution for a few weeks. This allows both partners to test out an idea without committing long-term.
- ***Split Decisions:*** If a compromise feels impossible, it may be helpful to agree to alternate decisions. For example, if one partner prefers to spend vacation time at the beach while the other prefers the mountains, consider alternating destinations each year.

4. Establish a Dialogue of Acceptance

In some cases, it may be necessary to agree to disagree. When an issue is deeply entrenched and both partners have made genuine efforts to understand each other's perspectives, it can be healthy to accept that not all conflicts will have a resolution. This dialogue of acceptance does not mean giving up; rather, it signifies a mutual understanding and respect for each other's differences.

To create this dialogue:

- Acknowledge the Importance of the Issue: Each partner should validate the other's feelings and recognize the significance of the issue at hand.
- Express Gratitude: Thank each other for being willing to engage in difficult conversations, even if the issue remains unresolved.

5. Consider Professional Help

If gridlock persists despite your best efforts, seeking the assistance of a qualified therapist or counselor can provide valuable support. A professional can offer new perspectives and techniques for navigating challenging issues, and facilitate productive communication between partners. Therapy can also provide a safe space for couples to explore deep-seated feelings and past experiences that may be contributing to gridlock.

Overcoming conflict gridlock requires patience, understanding, and a willingness to engage in open dialogue. By recognizing the signs of gridlock, understanding the underlying issues, and employing strategies such as curiosity, shared goals, compromises, and acceptance, couples can work together to break free from the cycle of frustration. While not every conflict will be resolved, fostering a sense of partnership and mutual respect allows couples to strengthen their relationship and deepen their emotional connection. With commitment and effort, couples can transform gridlock into an opportunity for growth, ultimately leading to a more resilient and fulfilling marriage.

Understanding Perpetual Issues and Long-Term Conflicts

In every marriage, some disagreements persist over time, resurfacing in various forms no matter how often they're addressed. These are known as "perpetual issues." Unlike solvable problems, which can be resolved through dialogue and compromise, perpetual issues are often rooted in deep-seated values, beliefs, and individual differences. Understanding these perpetual issues is crucial for navigating long-term conflicts in a way that promotes harmony and connection.

What Are Perpetual Issues?

Perpetual issues typically stem from fundamental differences in personality, upbringing, or lifestyle preferences. They can encompass a wide range of topics, including:

- *Money Management:* Differing views on spending, saving, and financial priorities.
- *Child-Rearing Practices:* Conflicting ideas about discipline, education, and lifestyle choices for children.
- *Household Responsibilities:* Disagreements about the division of labor, cleanliness, and organization.
- *Lifestyle Preferences:* Clashing preferences for social activities, leisure time, or work-life balance.

These issues can feel cyclical and unresolvable, leading couples to feel frustrated and defeated. However, understanding and managing these conflicts can transform them from sources of tension into opportunities for deeper connection and acceptance.

Recognizing the Nature of Perpetual Issues

The first step in managing perpetual issues is recognizing their nature. Unlike solvable problems that can be addressed with practical solutions, perpetual issues often remain unresolved over the long term. This realization can be both liberating and daunting. It helps couples understand that it's not a failure of their relationship but a reflection of their differences.

Key Characteristics of Perpetual Issues:

- They Don't Have a Clear Solution: No matter how many times couples discuss these issues, a definitive resolution may never be reached.
- They Often Resurface: Perpetual issues tend to come back into conversation, especially during times of stress or conflict.
- They Are Linked to Core Values: These conflicts often relate to what each partner values most, making them deeply personal.

1. Embrace Acceptance

Understanding that perpetual issues are a normal part of any marriage can help couples embrace acceptance. Acceptance involves recognizing that both partners are unlikely to change their fundamental beliefs or preferences. Instead of focusing on winning the argument or changing the other person's mind, couples should focus on accepting their differences. This mindset fosters a more compassionate and understanding environment.

How to Embrace Acceptance:
- Acknowledge Your Differences: Regularly remind each other that differences are a natural part of any relationship.
- Practice Self-Reflection: Reflect on your own beliefs and how they shape your perspective on the issue at hand.
- Share Your Feelings: Communicate openly about how the issue impacts you, without placing blame.

2. Focus on Emotional Connection

While perpetual issues may never be resolved, couples can still cultivate a strong emotional connection by focusing on the relationship itself. Building intimacy through shared experiences, open communication, and mutual respect can create a foundation that withstands the challenges posed by perpetual conflicts.

Ways to Enhance Emotional Connection:
- Prioritize Quality Time: Spend time together engaging in activities that strengthen your bond, whether it's date nights, hobbies, or simply sharing daily experiences.
- Communicate Regularly: Maintain open lines of communication, discussing feelings, needs, and any new developments related to the issue.
- Express Gratitude: Regularly express appreciation for each other, recognizing the effort both partners put into navigating conflicts.

3. Establish Ground Rules for Discussions

When engaging in conversations about perpetual issues, it's essential to establish ground rules to ensure respectful dialogue. Creating a safe space for discussion helps prevent escalation and allows both partners to express themselves without fear of judgment.

Effective Ground Rules:
- No Blame or Criticism: Focus on expressing feelings and perspectives rather than attacking your partner.
- Stay on Topic: Avoid bringing up unrelated issues or past grievances during the discussion.
- Set a Time Limit: Establish a time frame for discussions to avoid prolonged arguments that can lead to frustration.

4. Find Common Ground
Even when dealing with perpetual issues, there are often areas of agreement or common ground. Identifying shared values can help couples navigate conflicts more effectively and create a sense of teamwork.

Strategies for Finding Common Ground:
- Identify Shared Goals: Discuss the underlying goals or desires associated with the issue. For example, both partners may want financial security, even if their approaches differ.
- Explore Compromise: While some aspects may remain non-negotiable, explore where both partners can make concessions to meet each other halfway.

- Celebrate Small Wins: Acknowledge any progress made, no matter how small, in addressing the issue or finding ways to coexist with it.

5. Maintain Perspective

Finally, it's essential to maintain perspective when dealing with perpetual issues. Understand that no relationship is without challenges, and the goal is not perfection but rather a loving partnership that accommodates differences.

Maintaining Perspective:
- Reflect on Your Relationship: Regularly remind yourselves of the love, connection, and shared experiences that define your partnership.
- Recognize Growth: Acknowledge how you have both grown as individuals and as a couple, even when faced with ongoing challenges.
- Focus on the Positive: Shift the focus from the perpetual issue to the strengths of your relationship. Celebrate the qualities that brought you together in the first place.

Perpetual issues are an inevitable part of any long-term relationship. By understanding their nature, embracing acceptance, focusing on emotional connection, establishing ground rules for discussions, finding common ground, and maintaining perspective, couples can navigate these long-term conflicts with grace and understanding. While some disagreements may never reach a resolution, the ability to coexist with these differences can foster a deeper sense of intimacy and respect, ultimately strengthening the marriage.

By approaching perpetual issues as opportunities for growth rather than obstacles, couples can create a resilient and fulfilling partnership that withstands the test of time.

Conflict Management Strategies

Conflict is an inevitable part of any relationship, especially in marriage. Differences in opinions, values, and needs can lead to misunderstandings and disagreements. However, how couples manage these conflicts can significantly influence the health and longevity of their relationship. Employing effective conflict management strategies can turn potentially damaging situations into opportunities for growth, deeper understanding, and stronger connections. Here are several strategies that couples can use to navigate conflicts constructively.

1. Establish Open Communication

Effective communication is the cornerstone of conflict resolution. Establishing a safe and open environment for discussion encourages both partners to express their thoughts and feelings without fear of judgment. Here are some key components of open communication:

Active Listening: Make a conscious effort to truly listen to your partner. This means not only hearing their words but also understanding their feelings and perspectives. Use verbal and non-verbal cues to show engagement, such as nodding, maintaining eye contact, and summarizing what they've said.

Expressing Feelings Clearly: Use "I" statements to communicate feelings without placing blame. For example, say

"I feel hurt when you don't acknowledge my efforts" rather than "You never appreciate what I do." This approach reduces defensiveness and fosters understanding.

2. Identify the Root Cause of the Conflict

Often, the surface issue is not the true cause of the conflict. To resolve the disagreement effectively, both partners must dig deeper to understand the underlying emotions and needs driving their responses. Take time to reflect on questions such as:

What am I truly feeling?

What are the unmet needs behind my feelings?

How do past experiences influence my perspective on this issue?

By addressing the root cause, couples can work together to find solutions that satisfy both partners' needs.

3. Stay Calm and Manage Emotions

Conflicts can trigger strong emotions, which can cloud judgment and escalate the situation. It's essential to stay calm and manage emotions during discussions. Here are some strategies to help maintain composure:

Take Breaks: If emotions run high, take a timeout to cool down. Agree on a specific time to reconvene the discussion, allowing both partners to process their feelings and return to the conversation with a clearer mindset.

Practice Deep Breathing: Engage in deep breathing exercises to calm your nervous system. Take slow, deep breaths to help ground yourself and reduce feelings of anxiety or anger.

4. Focus on Solutions, Not Blame

When conflicts arise, it can be easy to slip into a blame game, which only exacerbates the situation. Instead, shift the focus from assigning blame to finding solutions. Here's how:

Collaborative Problem-Solving: Approach conflicts as a team. Instead of viewing the situation as a win-lose scenario, work together to identify potential solutions that satisfy both partners' needs. Use phrases like "How can we work together to solve this?" to foster collaboration.

Be Open to Compromise: Compromise involves both partners giving up something to reach a mutually acceptable solution.

Be willing to make concessions, as this demonstrates respect for your partner's needs and fosters a spirit of cooperation.

5. Set Ground Rules for Disagreements

Establishing ground rules for discussions can create a respectful and productive environment. These rules help both partners feel safe and valued during conflicts. Consider implementing the following guidelines:

- ***No Personal Attacks:*** Agree to avoid insults, name-calling, or derogatory comments. Focus on the issue at hand, not the person.
- ***Time Limits:*** Set a time limit for discussions to prevent them from dragging on indefinitely. This encourages

both partners to express their views concisely and keeps the conversation focused.

- *No Interruptions:* Allow each partner to speak without interruption. This demonstrates respect for each other's opinions and encourages active listening.

6. Use Humor Wisely

When appropriate, humor can diffuse tension and lighten the mood during conflicts. A well-timed joke or light-hearted comment can help both partners feel more relaxed and open. However, it's essential to use humor carefully, ensuring that it doesn't come across as dismissive or sarcastic. The goal is to foster connection and ease rather than to trivialize the issue.

7. Seek Professional Support When Needed

Some conflicts may be too deep-rooted or complex for couples to resolve on their own. If conflicts persist despite your best efforts, consider seeking the support of a qualified therapist or counselor. Professional guidance can provide new insights, tools, and techniques for managing conflicts more effectively.

8. Reflect and Learn from Conflicts

After navigating a conflict, take time to reflect on the experience. Consider what worked well, what could be improved, and how both partners can grow from the experience. This reflective practice can help couples learn from their conflicts and develop healthier patterns of interaction in the future.

Conflict is a natural part of any relationship, but it doesn't have to be destructive. By implementing effective conflict management strategies—such as open communication, identifying root causes, staying calm, focusing on solutions, setting ground rules, using humor wisely, seeking professional support, and reflecting on experiences—couples can navigate conflicts in a way that strengthens their bond and fosters deeper understanding. Rather than viewing conflicts as obstacles, embrace them as opportunities for growth, connection, and a more resilient partnership. With commitment and effort, couples can transform challenges into catalysts for a deeper and more fulfilling relationship.

Chapter 7: Create Shared Meaning

In a successful marriage, both partners not only navigate conflicts and celebrate joys but also build a shared sense of purpose and meaning. This chapter delves into the importance of creating shared meaning in a relationship, exploring how it fosters intimacy, strengthens connections, and provides a foundation for a fulfilling life together.

Understanding Shared Meaning

Shared meaning refers to the understanding and significance that partners ascribe to their life experiences, values, traditions, and aspirations. It encompasses the narratives couples create about their lives together, shaping their identity as a couple and influencing their interactions. Shared meaning acts as a glue that binds partners together, allowing them to navigate life's challenges with a sense of unity and purpose.

The Importance of Shared Meaning

Strengthens Emotional Bonds: When partners share meaning in their experiences and goals, they develop a deeper emotional connection. This bond fosters trust, loyalty, and intimacy, making it easier to weather life's storms together.

Enhances Communication: A shared narrative encourages open and honest communication. Couples who understand each other's values and dreams can discuss their thoughts and feelings more freely, reducing misunderstandings and increasing empathy.

Provides a Sense of Direction: Shared meaning creates a common vision for the future. Couples who work together toward shared goals are more likely to feel a sense of purpose and fulfillment in their relationship.

Promotes Resilience: When couples face challenges, a shared sense of meaning can serve as a source of strength. It reminds partners of their commitment to each other and the life they are building together, helping them navigate difficulties with a united front.

Building Shared Meaning

Creating shared meaning requires intentional effort and a willingness to engage in deep conversations. Here are several strategies to help couples cultivate shared meaning in their relationship:

1. Explore Values and Beliefs

Understanding each partner's core values and beliefs is essential for creating shared meaning. Schedule time to discuss what matters most to each of you, such as family, career, spirituality, and personal growth. Ask questions like:

- What values do you want to instill in our family?
- How do our individual beliefs shape our decisions?
- What traditions or practices are important to you?

Through these conversations, couples can identify overlapping values and build a shared foundation that reflects their combined beliefs.

2. Create Shared Rituals and Traditions

Rituals and traditions play a significant role in building shared meaning. They create moments of connection and continuity in a relationship, reinforcing the couple's bond. Consider establishing rituals for daily, weekly, or yearly activities, such as:

- Daily Check-Ins: Take a few minutes each day to share highlights and challenges, fostering connection and communication.
- Weekly Date Nights: Prioritize time together to nurture your relationship and create special memories.
- Annual Family Traditions: Celebrate holidays or special occasions in a way that reflects both partners' values and fosters a sense of belonging.

These shared rituals help couples reinforce their identity as a team while creating lasting memories.

3. Engage in Meaningful Conversations

Deep, meaningful conversations are essential for fostering shared meaning. These discussions allow couples to explore their dreams, fears, and aspirations, creating a richer understanding of each other. Aim to engage in conversations that go beyond surface-level topics, addressing:

- *Future goals and dreams:* What do you envision for our lives together?

- **Personal passions and interests:** How can we support each other in pursuing our individual goals?
- *Family dynamics and expectations:* How do we want to navigate family relationships together?

Being open and vulnerable in these conversations deepens emotional intimacy and lays the groundwork for shared meaning.

4. Collaborate on Goals and Dreams

Shared meaning flourishes when couples work together toward common goals and dreams. Discuss both short-term and long-term aspirations, including:

- *Career Goals:* How can you support each other's professional aspirations?
- *Family Planning:* What are your hopes for children, and what values do you want to impart to them?
- *Personal Growth:* How can you encourage each other's individual growth and development?

By collaborating on these goals, couples create a shared vision for their future, reinforcing their commitment to one another.

5. Celebrate Achievements Together

Acknowledging and celebrating milestones—big and small—contributes to a sense of shared meaning. Recognize your achievements as a couple, such as:

- Completing a home project
- Reaching a financial goal
- Overcoming a challenge together

Celebrating these moments reinforces the idea that you are working toward shared success, strengthening your emotional bond.

Navigating Differences in Meaning

It's essential to recognize that differences in meaning can arise, and that's perfectly normal. Each partner brings their own perspectives and experiences to the relationship. When conflicts arise around shared meaning, it's important to approach these differences with curiosity and respect. *Here are some strategies to navigate differing perspectives:*

- *Practice Empathy:* Try to understand your partner's point of view, even if you don't agree. Ask questions to gain insight into their feelings and experiences.
- *Negotiate Compromise:* Find ways to integrate both partners' values and beliefs into shared practices. This may involve creating new traditions or rituals that honor both perspectives.
- *Stay Open-Minded:* Be willing to explore and adapt your understanding of shared meaning as your relationship evolves. Life circumstances and individual growth can change the way you both perceive meaning.

Creating shared meaning is a vital component of a successful marriage. By exploring values, establishing rituals, engaging in meaningful conversations, collaborating on goals, and celebrating achievements, couples can deepen their connection and build a strong foundation for their relationship. While differences in meaning may arise, approaching these conflicts with empathy and open-mindedness allows couples to navigate challenges while fostering intimacy and understanding. Ultimately, shared meaning enriches the marriage, providing a sense of direction and purpose that enhances the couple's journey together.

Creating a Shared Vision and Purpose

A strong marriage is built on a shared vision and purpose that aligns both partners toward common goals and aspirations. When couples have a unified direction, they not only navigate life's challenges more effectively, but they also experience a deeper connection and sense of fulfillment in their relationship. Creating this shared vision involves understanding each partner's dreams, values, and expectations, and then weaving these elements into a cohesive plan for the future.

1. Define Your Individual Visions

The first step in creating a shared vision is for each partner to articulate their individual dreams and aspirations. Set aside time for open and honest discussions about what you envision for your life, career, family, and personal growth. Consider asking each other questions like:

- What are your long-term goals?
- What kind of lifestyle do you aspire to have?
- How do you see our family evolving in the future?

Encouraging each other to share these personal visions fosters deeper understanding and respect for each other's hopes and desires.

2. Identify Common Values

Once each partner has shared their individual visions, the next step is to identify common values that resonate with both of you. Discuss the principles that guide your lives and decisions, such as honesty, kindness, adventure, or financial stability. Finding shared values creates a foundation for your shared vision and helps ensure that both partners feel aligned in their aspirations.

3. Craft a Unified Vision Statement

With a clear understanding of your individual visions and shared values, it's time to create a unified vision statement for your marriage. This statement serves as a guiding light, reminding both partners of their goals and the life they are building together. It can include elements such as:

- ***Goals for the Future:*** What do you want to achieve together in the coming years?
- ***Family Dynamics:*** What type of family culture do you wish to cultivate?
- ***Lifestyle Choices:*** How do you want to live your lives, and what experiences do you want to prioritize?

Writing this statement together and placing it somewhere visible in your home can serve as a constant reminder of your shared purpose.

Using Rituals and Traditions to Strengthen Your Bond

Rituals and traditions play a crucial role in reinforcing the shared vision and purpose within a marriage. These practices create a sense of continuity and connection, allowing couples to celebrate their relationship while fostering emotional intimacy.

1. Establish Daily Rituals

Daily rituals can help couples maintain a strong bond amidst the hustle and bustle of life. Simple practices, such as:

- **Morning Check-Ins:** Start each day by sharing your intentions and goals for the day.
- **Dinner Together:** Make it a priority to share meals together, allowing time for conversation and connection.
- **Bedtime Reflections**: At the end of the day, take a few moments to reflect on what went well and express gratitude for each other.

These daily rituals promote open communication and help couples remain attuned to each other's feelings and needs.

2. Create Weekly or Monthly Traditions

In addition to daily rituals, establishing weekly or monthly traditions can enhance the sense of togetherness. These might include:

- **Date Nights:** Dedicate one night a week to each other, whether it's a fancy dinner out or a cozy movie night at home.
- **Family Activities**: Plan regular family outings or game nights that reinforce family bonds and create cherished memories.
- **Goal-Setting Sessions**: Set aside time to revisit your shared vision, discuss progress, and adjust your goals as needed.

These traditions provide opportunities for connection and collaboration, reinforcing the shared purpose within your marriage.

3. Celebrate Milestones and Achievements
Acknowledging and celebrating milestones is a powerful way to strengthen your bond and affirm your shared vision. This could involve:

- *Anniversary Celebrations:* Commemorate your wedding anniversary with special rituals or trips that reflect your journey together.
- *Goal Achievements:* Celebrate when you reach significant goals as a couple, whether it's a home purchase, a promotion, or a personal milestone.
- *Family Traditions:* Establish family traditions for holidays, birthdays, or other special occasions that reflect your shared values and create lasting memories.

These celebrations foster a sense of accomplishment and togetherness, reinforcing the importance of your shared journey.

Creating a shared vision and purpose, combined with the use of rituals and traditions, strengthens the bond between partners in a marriage. By defining individual dreams, identifying common values, and crafting a unified vision statement, couples can cultivate a deeper understanding of their shared aspirations. Additionally, establishing daily rituals, creating weekly traditions, and celebrating milestones help reinforce the emotional connection that sustains a fulfilling relationship. By investing in these practices, couples can navigate life's challenges with resilience and create a lasting partnership rooted in love, respect, and shared meaning.

Conclusion:

Your Journey to a Happier Marriage.

Starting on the path to a happier marriage requires a commitment to growth, understanding, and communication. It is a continual process that involves effort, patience, and a willingness to accept both the benefits and drawbacks of collaboration. Applying the principles outlined in this book—enhancing your love maps, developing fondness and admiration, turning toward each other, allowing influence, solving solvable problems, overcoming conflict gridlock, and creating shared meaning—can help you foster a deeper, more fulfilling relationship with your partner.

Embrace Growth together.

A happy marriage is not a destination, but rather an ongoing process of growth and discovery. It is critical to approach a relationship with an open heart and mind, accepting that both partners will change with time. Accept these shifts as an opportunity to strengthen your relationship and understanding. Revisit your shared vision and goals on a regular basis, making adjustments as needed to reflect your changing requirements and aspirations.

Communicate openly and honestly.

Effective communication is crucial to the success of any marriage. Prioritize open and honest interactions with your partner, creating an environment in which both of you feel comfortable expressing your opinions and feelings. Actively listen, validate each other's emotions, and swiftly correct any misconceptions. Remember that communication is more than just exchanging words; it is about creating a genuine connection that develops your friendship.

cultivate respect and appreciation.
Respect and admiration are essential components of a healthy marriage. Make it a habit to express gratitude for your partner's efforts, no matter how big or small. Recognize their accomplishments and efforts, and appreciate their uniqueness. By instilling a culture of respect and gratitude, you create a nurturing environment in which both partners may thrive.

Navigate Challenges with Resilience.
Every marriage will confront difficulties, whether they stem from external conditions or internal problems. The key to a good partnership is how you work through these issues together. Use positive conflict resolution tactics, approach differences with empathy, and seek solutions rather than assigning blame. When faced with barriers, remember that you are a team working toward a same objective, and supporting one another through difficulties only strengthens your bond.

Invest in your relationship.
A happy marriage, like every other valuable effort, takes investment. Make an intentional effort to prioritize your relationship in the face of life's responsibilities. Make time for date nights, family rituals, and shared activities that promote

closeness. Engage in continuous learning about one another, experiencing new interests and experiences together. The more you invest in your relationship, the more fulfilling it will be.

The Path Ahead

Remember that each relationship is unique as you embark on this journey to a healthier marriage. There is no one-size-fits-all approach, but by adhering to the ideals of love, respect, and understanding, you may build a long-lasting partnership. Accept the ups and downs, and treasure the moments of joy and connection along the road.

To summarize, your journey to a healthier marriage is both personal and shared, formed by your specific circumstances, values, and goals. By accepting progress, communicating openly, fostering respect, overcoming obstacles with perseverance, and investing in your relationship, you are laying the groundwork for a healthy, long-lasting partnership. Remember that happiness in marriage is not a destination; it is a lovely journey you take together, full of love, laughter, and shared significance. Here's to your journey—one of discovery, joy, and lasting love.